Foreword

Tuina was the evolvement of cuneiform stone remedy in the Neolithic. It was called Anmo (or Anqiao, or Daoyin) before the Ming Dynasty (1368-1644) because of its simple techniques and nonsystematic theory. After the Ming Dynasty, with the development of traditional Chinese medicine theory, which was continuously infiltrating into the tuina therapy field and guiding the clinical treatment with an obvious increase in effect, tuinaology was therefore formed. Ever since its initiation, it already has had a history of several thousands of years. In today's society, science and technology are developing rapidly. In order to popularize, develop and make best use of the traditional Chinese medicine for the human being health, it is of great significance to publish this book in English.

It should meet the demands of the speedy development of modern civilized society to popularize the tuinaology of traditional Chinese medicine, so that people can get more harvest with less time. Therefore, the first characteristic of this book is terse and concise as the tuina techniques adopted in the treatment are demonstrated with illustration of simple diagrams instead of narrative words, so readers can learn it with ease. The second characteristic is separate and independent. The diagrams of tuina techniques demonstration are separately used in each disease and independently laid out to the other diseases, thus readers can get double achievements with half effort, dispensing with the restlessness of spending lots of energy and time in consultation of tuina techniques all over the book.

To develop tuinaology cannot just stay on the general treatment, for it will lead to the simplification, mediocrity and irregularity of tuina, which mean anyone can manage it without theoretic guidance, apply it without the consideration of differentiation, time and places, and do it irregularly according to one's own way. The right way to proceed is that we should discuss and analyze the principles, symptoms and effects of treatment on tuina in simple but clear language, so as to let the readers grasp it within a short period of time and increase the proficiency by analogy. So the third characteristic of this book is popular and practicable. It is a combination of traditional Chinese medicine theory and clinical practice of tuina techniques. It is written in a form easy to learn and remember. In this case, it is not only good for the readers to quickly understand the characteristics of each technique, treatment principles and the indications, but also favorable to guide the readers to put what they have learned into clinical treatment.

It is not a matter of one morning or evening to totally master the tuinaology and flexibly apply the techniques of tuina on the treatment of diseases, especially the techniques requiring "moving but not superficial, forceful but not stagnated." Therefore, attention should be paid to the following precautions while reading the book.

1. Accuracy of the points. In the book, the location of each point is precisely elaborated and indicated. If readers are still not clear about the anatomic positions of the points, please consult firstly the sketch figures of points and proportional measurements at the beginning of the book, or other professional books concerning acupoints, so as to achieve a satisfactory treatment effect. Generally speaking, if the book says "place a finger on one particular point," this will require the massager accurately massage on this point; if the book says "place four fingers (or one palm or sole) on (or push to) some point," this will require the massager's fingers (or palm or sole) to be placed at (or pushed to) the same height of this point or the region of the point.

2. Measurement of the points. The *cun* mentioned in the book refers to the unit adopted by proportional measurement and finger measurement. Details can be seen in the figures of Bone-Length Measurement and Commonly Used Points at the appendix of the book. Besides, in order to provide more convenience for the readers in reading the book, the location of the same point is explained differently in the diagrams of different tuina techniques. For example, in one technique diagram, which shows the massage of Shenque (CV 8) and Guanyuan (CV 4) points, it is written that the location of Shenque (CV 8) is at the center of the umbilicus and the location of Guanyuan (CV 4) is 3 *cun* directly below Shenque (CV 8). But in another technique diagram showing massage of Qugu (CV 2) and Guanyuan (CV 4) points, it is said that the location of Qugu (CV 2) is at the middle point of the upper margin of pubic bone and the location of Guanyuan (CV 4) now is 2 *cun* above Qugu (CV 2). In this way, readers will get a clear idea about each technique just by taking a glance at the corresponding diagram of points.

3. Lasting time and frequency of tuina techniques. The quintessence of traditional Chinese medicine is the conception of the organism as a whole as well as diagnosis and treatment based on an overall analysis of symptoms and signs, the cause, nature and location of the illness and the patient's physical condition. Different patient has different physical condition, pathological status and prognosis, so the same tuina technique applying on the different patients requires alternation in length of operating time and frequency. The massager should appropriately prolong or reduce the manipulating time within certain limitation so as to get a satisfactory treatment effect.

4. Degrees of strength and dexterity of tuina techniques. Only with proper

Practical Chinese Tuina Therapy with Illustrations

Written by Pan Chang
Translated by Li Yachan

NEW WORLD PRESS BEIJING, CHINA

First Edition 1998

Edited by Wang Jianying
Book design by Li Hui

ISBN 7-80005-414-4/R•039

Published by
NEW WORLD PRESS
24 Baiwanzhuang Road, Beijing 100037, China

Distributed by
CHINA INTERNATIONAL BOOK TRADING CORPORATION
35 Chegongzhuang Xilu, Beijing 100044, China
P.O. Box 399, Beijing, China

Printed in the People's Republic of China

tuina strength from the massager, can the satisfactory treatment effect be achieved. So the intensity of strength exerted in the treatment is not proportional to the treatment effect. In some case, it is opposite. Moreover, the dexterity is even more important. To pursuit an excellent skill on tuina, the massager not only needs to study hard and practice more, but also needs to learn *qigong* to increase his internal power, so that he can be dexterous, not clumsy in the tuina treatment. On the other hand, if a reader wants to be a qualified Tuina therapist, he should not only learn the theory of traditional Chinese medicine, but also needs to know some theory of western medicine, such as pathology, physiology and anatomy, etc. Thus, he will know which pattern of a disease can be treated by tuina, and that if the same disease showing different clinical symptoms, it may be no longer treated by Tuina. He also will know what the tuina treatment effects are and whether the tuina regions and point locations are correct or not, etc.

At the moment of publication of this book (English version), I would like to extend my lofty greetings to my teachers Prof. Luo Jinghong and Prof. Luo Zhongda, who warmly supported and encouraged me to write this book; and I also would like to express my gratitude to all my family members, who have shown deep considerations for me and offered hearty assistance in my research of traditional Chinese medicine for a long time.

I welcome colleagues, home and abroad, to comment on the text. The comment will be beneficial for future revision of this book so that it will serve as a book for popularizing the traditional Chinese medicine, to meet the demands of popularization and development of traditional Chinese medicine in the better way.

CONTENTS

Chronic Gastritis

Clinical Manifestations

This comprises a group of indigestion symptoms, for example, uncomfortable feeling in the upper abdomen, belching with acid regurgitation, nausea and vomiting, poor appetite, etc. Some patients may present chronic upper abdominal pain of differing degrees of severity, which are located diffusely on the left side of the upper abdomen, involving a wide area rather than local and fixed pain.

Differentiation of syndromes:

A. Retention of food type: Distention and stuffiness in gastric region, in severe cases gastric pain, acid regurgitation and vomiting, the pain being alleviated after vomiting, pale tongue with thick and sticky coating, rolling pulse.

B. Accumulation of heat in the stomach type: Distention and fullness in gastric region, distending pain radiating to the hypochondriac regions, belching and constipation, red tongue with yellow coating, wiry and rapid pulse.

C. Stomach Yang deficiency type: Dull pain in gastric region with clear and thin fluid regurgitation, preference of warmth and pressure, poor appetite, cold extremities, loose stool, pale tongue with thin coating, soft and weak pulse.

D. Cold retention in the stomach type: Sudden onset of violent pain in gastric region, dislike of cold and preferring warmth, absence of thirst or preferring hot drinks, pale tongue with white and sticky coating, tense pulse.

Treatment Principle

Regulating *qi* and invigorating the spleen, removing the stagnation and relieving pain.

Tuina Techniques

A. Rubbing and pressing techniques on the upper abdomen.

B. Pushing technique on the upper abdomen.

C. Circular kneading technique on periumbilical region.

D. Conducting *qi* technique.

E. Small relieving *qi* stagnation technique.

F. Stationary circular pressing technique on Zusanli (ST 36).

G. Fist circular pressing technique on the back.

Addition or Subtraction Techniques

A. Retention of food type:

Addition: Chest stretching technique.

Subtraction: Circular kneading technique on periumbilical region.

B. Accumulation of heat in the stomach type:

Addition: 1. Rubbing and pressing techniques on the hypochondrium. 2. Digital pressing technique on the chest and abdomen. 3. Kneading and pressing techniques around the knee joint.

Subtraction: 1. Rubbing and pressing techniques on the upper abdomen. 2. Circular kneading technique on periumbilical region.

C. Stomach Yang deficiency type:

Addition: Squeezing and pushing techniques on the back.

D. Cold retention in the stomach type:

Addition: 1. Pressing technique along the midline of the abdomen. 2. Transverse rubbing technique across the umbilicus.

Subtraction: Rubbing and pressing techniques on the upper abdomen.

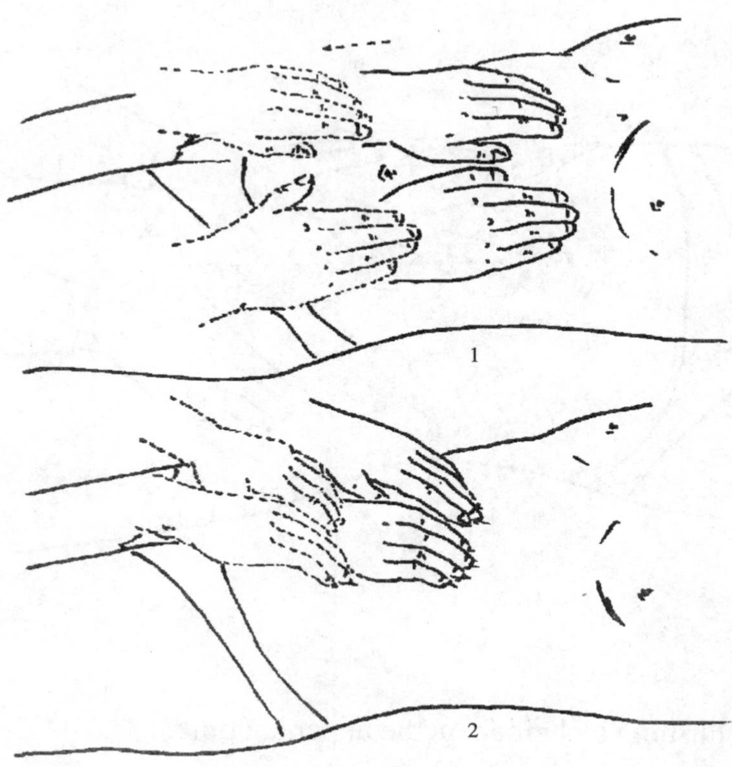

Rubbing and pressing techniques on the upper abdomen.

Manipulation

Place four finger-pulps of both hands on Burong (ST 19) and then rub downwards to Tianshu (ST 25). Repeat the massage for 1-2 minutes, then press Burong (ST 19) and Tianshu (ST 25) for 1-2 minutes.

Points

1. Burong (ST 19): 6 *cun* above the umbilicus and 2 *cun* lateral to the midline.
2. Tianshu (ST 25): 2 *cun* lateral to the center of the umbilicus.

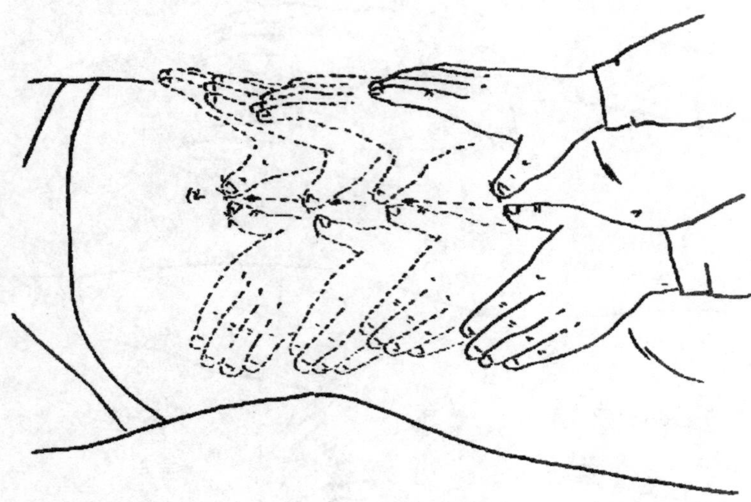

Pushing technique on the upper abdomen.

Manipulation

Place both thumbs on Jiuwei (CV 15) and let the other fingers fan out on both sides of the ribs. Conduct pushing and kneading techniques straight downwards past Zhongwan (CV 12), Xiawan (CV 10) and stop at Shuifen (CV 9). Repeat the manipulation for 3-5 minutes.

Points

1. Jiuwei (CV 15): Below the xiphoid process, 7 *cun* above the center of the umbilicus.

2. Zhongwan (CV 12): On the midline of the abdomen, 4 *cun* above the center of the umbilicus.

3. Xiawan (CV 10): On the midline of the abdomen, 2 *cun* above the center of the umbilicus.

4. Shuifen (CV 9): On the midline of the abdomen, 1 *cun* above the center of the umbilicus.

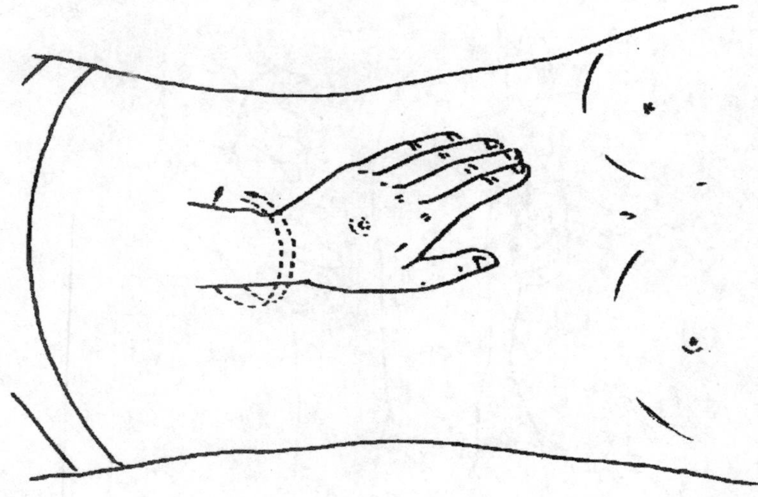

Circular kneading technique on periumbilical region.

Manipulation

Lay the center of a palm on Shenque (CV 8), knead the point clockwise and counterclockwise, in each direction the massage should last 2-3 minutes.

Points

Shenque (CV 8): In the center of the umbilicus.

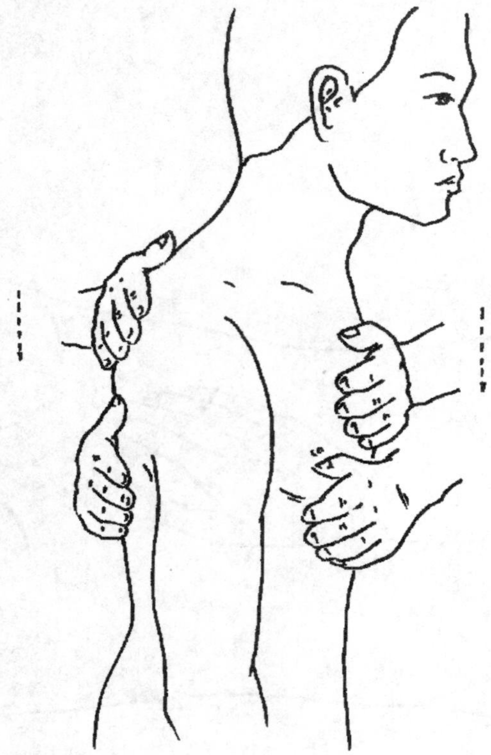

Conducting *qi* technique.

Manipulation

Place one palm on Xuanji (CV 21) on the middle of the chest and the other palm on Dazhui (GV 14) on the back. Massage downwards in rubbing technique following the anterior and posterior midlines and stop at Zhongting (CV 16) and Zhiyang (GV 9). Repeat the manipulation for 1-3 minutes.

Points

1. Xuanji (CV 21): On the anterior midline, at the midpoint of the sternal angle, at the level with the first intercostal space.

2. Dazhui (GV 14): Below the spinous process of the seventh cervical vertebra.

3. Zhongting (CV 16): On the midline of the sternum, at the level with the fifth intercostal space.

4. Zhiyang (GV 9): Below the spinous process of the seventh thoracic vertebra.

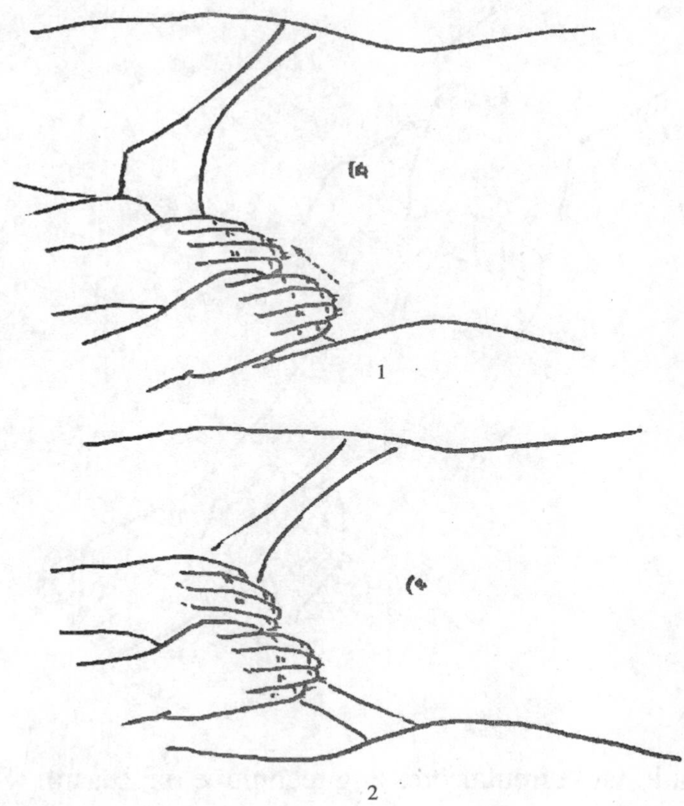

Small relieving *qi* stagnation technique.

Manipulation

Place four finger-pulps of both hands on unilateral Weidao (GB 28) located at the supramedial border of hip bone, rub and press in an inferior-medial direction and stop at Qichong (ST 30). Repeat the manipulation for 2-4 minutes.

Points

1. Weidao (GB 28): 1 *cun* anterior and inferior to the anterior superior iliac spine, about 3 *cun* lateral to the anterior midline.

2. Qichong (ST 30): 5 *cun* below and 2 *cun* lateral to the center of the umbilicus.

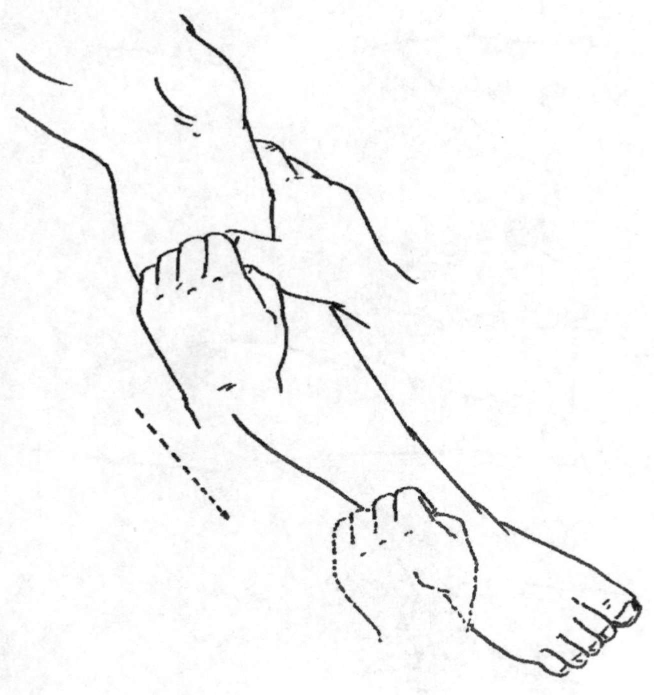

Stationary circular pressing technique on Zusanli (ST 36).

Manipulation

Place a thumb on Zusanli (ST 36) and knead the point. At the same time, flex four fingers of the other hand and place them on Yanglingquan (GB 34), then massage in pushing technique down to Xuanzhong (GB 39). Repeat the manipulation for 1-2 minutes.

Points

1. Zusanli (ST 36): One finger-breadth lateral to the anterior crest of the tibia, in m. tibialis anterior.

2. Yanglingquan (GB 34): In the depression anterior and inferior to the head of the fibula.

3. Xuanzhong (GB 39): 3 *cun* above the tip of the external malleolus, in the depression between the anterior border of the fibula and the tendons of m. peroneus longus and brevis.

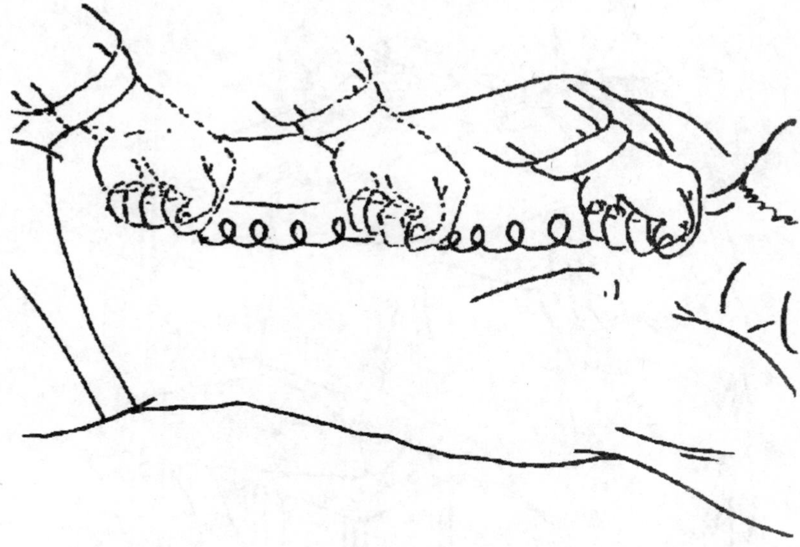

Fist circular pressing technique on the back.

Manipulation

Place fist knuckles of one hand on unilateral Dazhu (BL 11), knead downwards along one side of the spine past through Pishu (BL 20), Weishu (BL 21), Shenshu (BL 23), and stop at Dachangshu (BL 25). Treat both sides of the spine with this manipulation. Repeat on each side 2-5 minutes.

Points

1. Dazhu (BL 11): At the level of the lower border of the spinous process of the first thoracic vertebra and 1.5 *cun* lateral to the midline.

2. Pishu (BL 20): At the level of the lower border of the spinous process of the eleventh thoracic vertebra and 1.5 *cun* lateral to the midline.

3. Weishu (BL 21): At the level of the lower border of the spinous process of the twelfth thoracic vertebra and 1.5 *cun* lateral to the midline.

4. Shenshu (BL 23): At the level of the lower border of the spinous process of the second lumbar vertebra and 1.5 *cun* lateral to the midline.

5. Dazhangshu (BL 25): At the level of the lower border of the spinous process of the fourth lumbar vertebra and 1.5 *cun* lateral to the midline.

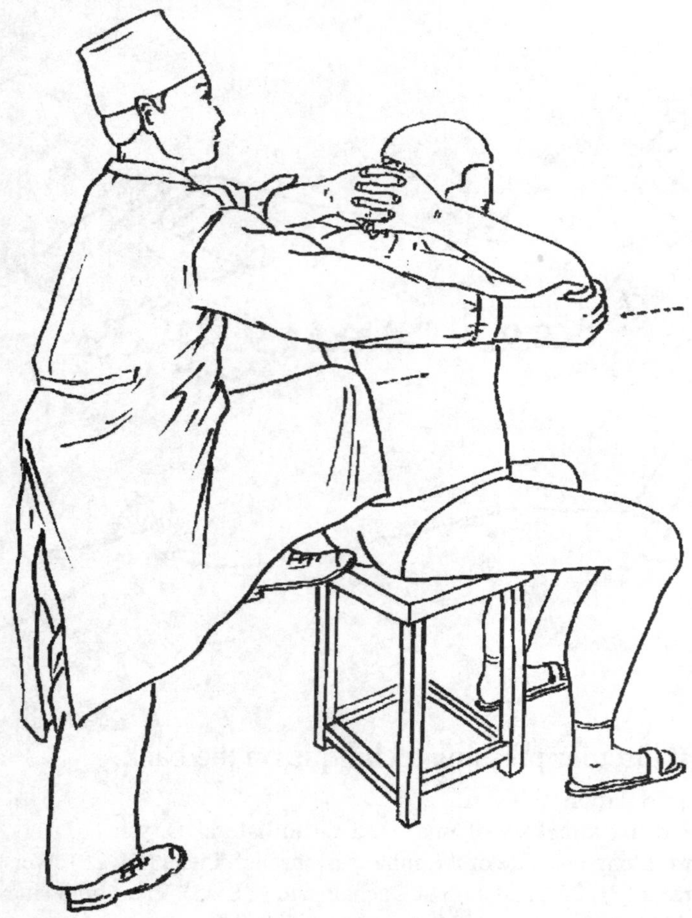

Chest stretching technique.

Manipulation

Let the hands go under the patient's armpits to the front, then wrap over and fix the patient's elbow regions. Place one knee on Taodao (GV 13) on patient's lower back. Instruct the patient to let his (her) chest stick out and take a deep breath. Slowly pull back the patient's elbows and let the knee push and press the back of the patient until the patient cannot inhale any more. Repeat the manipulation 3-5 times.

Points

Taodao (GV 13): Below the spinous process of the first thoracic vertebra.

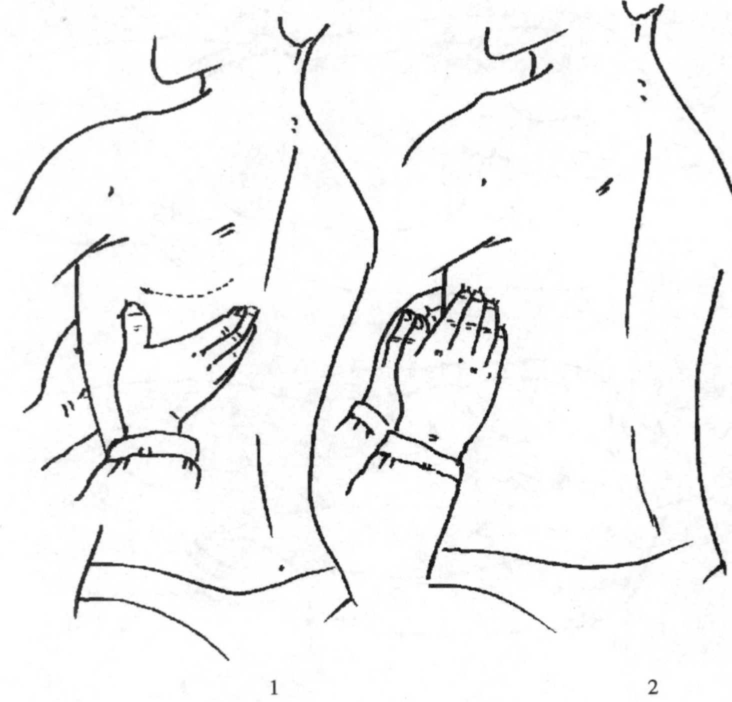

1 2

Rubbing and pressing techniques on the hypochondrium.

Manipulation

Place four finger-pulps of one hand on Burong (ST 19) and Chengman (ST 20). Place four finger-pulps of the other hand on Hunmen (BL 47) and Yanggang (BL 48) located on the opposite side. Press these points for 3-5 seconds. Then rub upward towards the axillary midline where the finger-pulps of both hands finally meet. Repeat the manipulation 1-3 minutes.

Points

1. Burong (ST 19): 6 *cun* above the umbilicus and 2 *cun* lateral to the midline.
2. Chengman (ST 20): 5 *cun* above the umbilicus and 2 *cun* lateral to the midline.
3. Hunmen (BL 47): At the level of the lower border of the spinous process of the ninth thoracic vertebra, 3 *cun* lateral to the midline.
4. Yanggang (BL 48): At the level of the lower border of the spinous process of the tenth thoracic vertebra, 3 *cun* lateral to the midline.

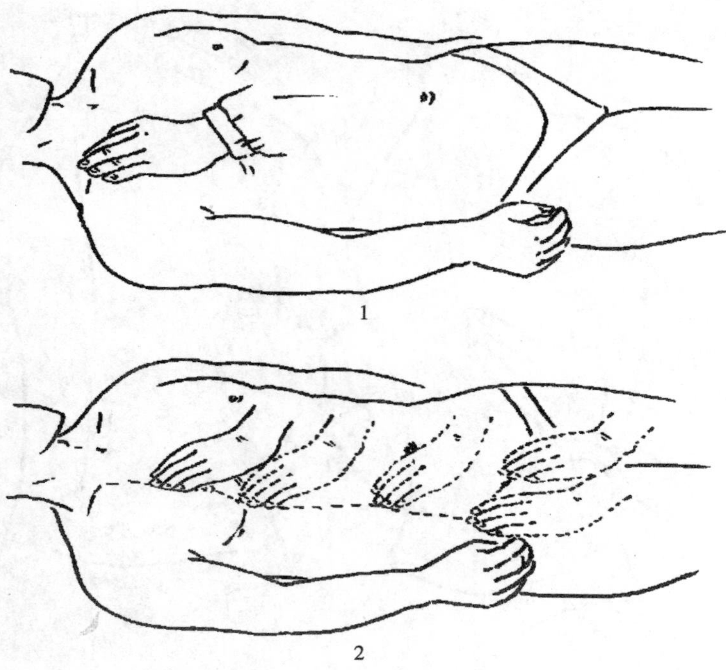

Digital pressing technique on chest and abdomen.

Manipulation

Place four fingertips of one hand on Qihu (ST 13), then slowly press the intercostal space downwards along Yingchuang (ST 16), Qimen (LR14), Daheng (SP 15), Fushe (SP 13), and stop at Qichong (ST 30). Repeat the manipulation 2-3 times.

Points

1. Qihu (ST 13): At the lower border of the middle of the clavicle, 4 *cun* lateral to the anterior midline.

2. Yingchuang (ST 16): In the third intercostal space, 4 *cun* lateral to the anterior midline.

3. Qimen (LR14): Directly below the nipple, in the sixth intercostal space.

4. Daheng (SP 15): 4 *cun* lateral to the center of the umbilicus.

5. Fushe (SP 13): 3.5 *cun* below the center of the umbilicus and 4 *cun* lateral to the anterior midline.

6. Qichong (ST 30): 5 *cun* below the center of the umbilicus and 2 *cun* lateral to the anterior midline.

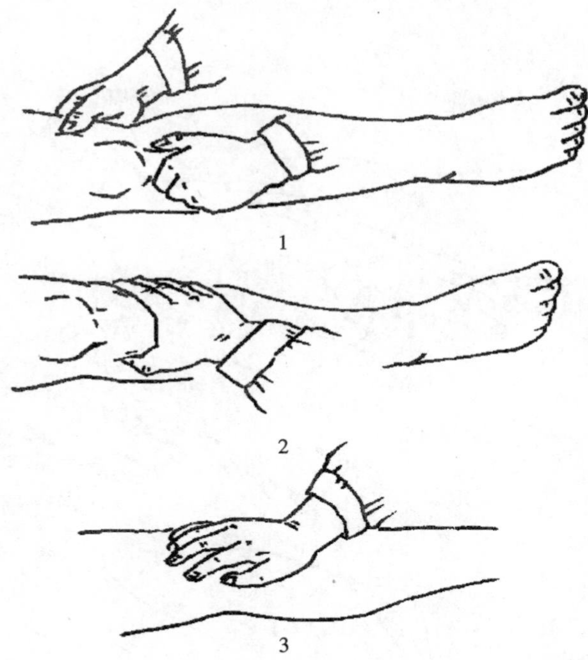

Kneading and pressing techniques around the knee joint.

Manipulation

1. Place the thumb of one hand on Xuehai (SP 10) and the thumb of the other hand and four fingertips on Neixiyan (Ex.LE4) and Waixiyan (ST 35) respectively. Press and knead the points simultaneously for 1-2 minutes.

2. Place the thumb and index finger of one hand on Yinlingquan (SP 9) and Yanglingquan (GB 34) respectively, then press and knead the points for 1-2 minutes.

3. Lastly, place one palm on kneecap, use four fingers to rub and pinch the area around the knee for 1-2 minutes.

Points

1. Xuehai (SP 10): 2 *cun* above the mediosuperior border of the patella.

2. Neixiyan (Ex.LE4): In the depression medial to the patellar ligament..

3. Waixiyan (ST 35): In the depression lateral to the tip of the patella.

4. Yinlingquan (SP 9): On the lower border of medial condyle of the tibia, in the depression on the medial border of the tibia.

5. Yanglingquan (GB 34): In the depression anterior and inferior to the head of the fibula.

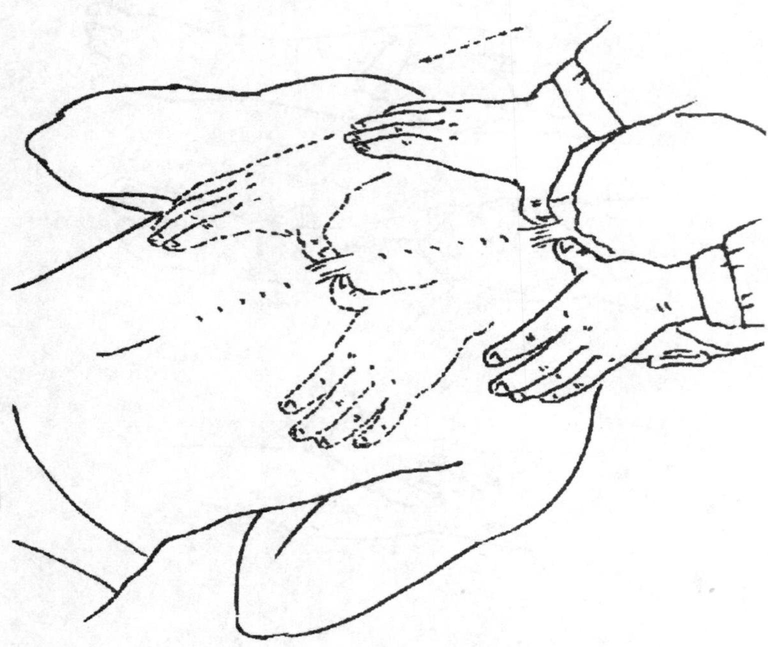

Squeezing and pushing techniques on the back.

Manipulation

With other fingers fanning out on each side of the back, place two thumb-pulps respectively on Dazhu (BL 11), then squeeze and push slowly at the back muscle along the spine, and stop at Geshu (BL 17). Repeat the manipulation for 3-5 minutes.

Points

1. Dazhu (BL 11): At the level of the lower border of the spinous process of the first thoracic vertebra and 1.5 *cun* lateral to the midline.

2. Geshu (BL 17): At the level of the lower border of the spinous process of the seventh thoracic vertebra and 1.5 *cun* lateral to the midline.

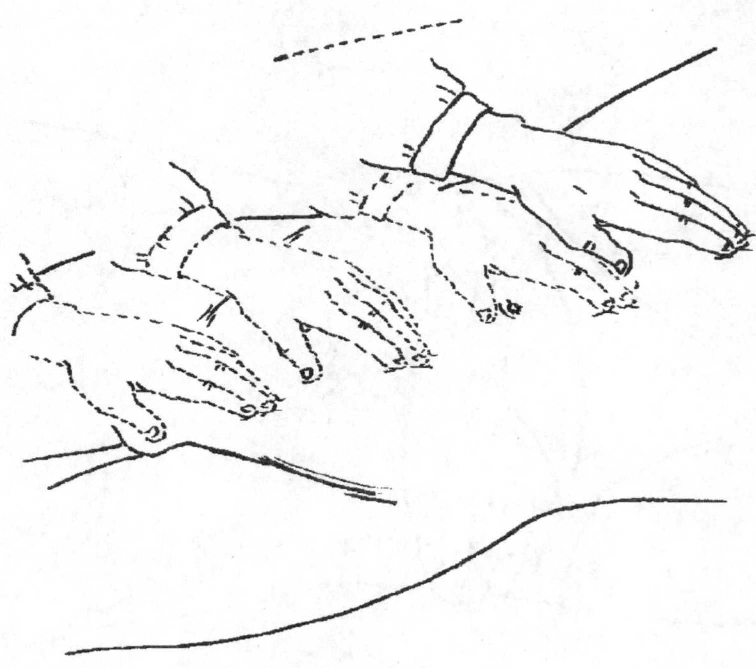

Pressing technique along the midline of the abdomen.

Manipulation

Place four fingertips of one hand on Shangwan (CV 13). Press straight downwards along the midline of the abdomen past Xiawan (CV 10), Guanyuan (CV 4) and stop at Qugu (CV 2). Repeat the manipulation for 1-3 minutes.

Points

1. Shangwan (CV 13): On the midline of the abdomen, 5 *cun* above the umbilicus.

2. Xiawan (CV 10): On the midline of the abdomen, 2 *cun* above the umbilicus.

3. Guanyuan (CV 4): On the midline of the abdomen, 3 *cun* below the umbilicus.

4. Qugu (CV 2): On the midline of the abdomen, 5 *cun* below the umbilicus.

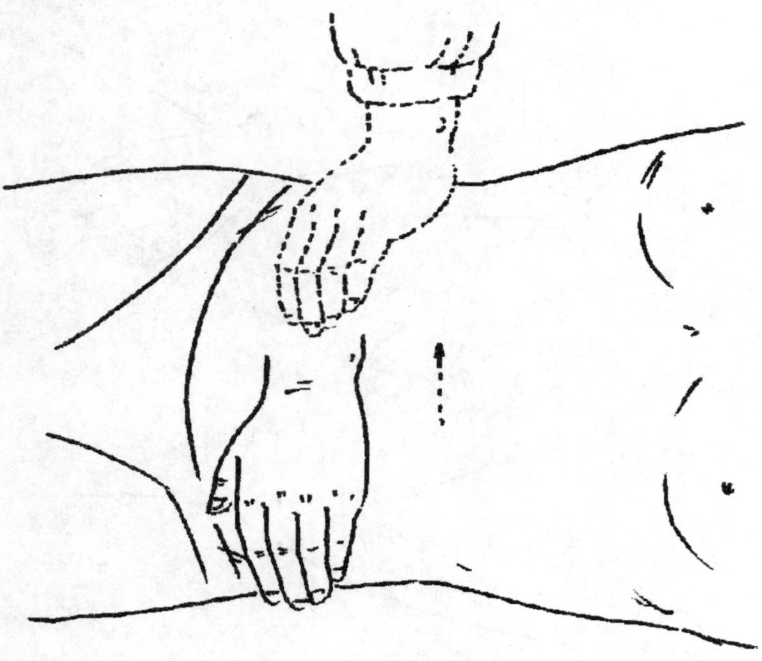

Transverse rubbing technique across the umbilicus.

Manipulation

Place four finger-pulps on one side of Daheng (SP 15) and Fujie (SP 14), rub transversely across the abdomen and past Tianshu (ST 25) and Wailing (ST 26) and stop at Daheng (SP 15) and Fujie (SP 14) on the opposite side. Repeat the manipulation for 2-3 minutes.

Points

1. Daheng (SP 15): 4 *cun* lateral to the center of the umbilicus.
2. Fujie (SP 14): 1.3 *cun* below the umbilicus and 4 *cun* lateral to the midline.
3. Tianshu (ST 25): 2 *cun* lateral to the center of the umbilicus.
4. Wailing (ST 26): 1 *cun* below the center of the umbilicus and 2 *cun* lateral to the midline.

Gastrointestinal Neurosis

Clinical Manifestations

There are gastrointestinal symptoms, such as chronic diarrhea or constipation, hiccup, acid regurgitation, etc., which are combined with headache, insomnia, lack of energy, poor memory, spontaneous or night sweating, aversion to cold in winter and to heat in summer.

Differentiation of syndromes:

A. Gastric neurosis is mainly manifested by gastric symptoms which can be divided into two types:

1. Spleen and stomach Yang deficiency type: Abdominal distention with poor appetite, dull pain in the upper abdomen alleviated by pressure, cold extremities, general lassitude and loose stool, associated with insomnia, dream-disturbed sleep and dislike of talking, pale tongue with white and slippery coating, deep and slow pulse.

2. Liver and spleen Yin deficiency type: Distention, stuffiness and wandering pain in the chest and hypochondrium, abdominal distention, poor appetite, loose stool, afternoon fever, associated with sighing, irritability and restlessness. Red tongue with scanty coating, wiry, thready and rapid pulse.

B. Intestinal neurosis is mainly manifested by intestinal symptoms which can be classified into two types:

1. *Qi* obstruction with abdominal pain type: Distending pain in the hypochondriac region, either on the left side or the right side, abdominal pain, poor appetite, irregular defecation, accompanied by restlessness and insomnia, pale tongue with thin and sticky coating, wiry pulse.

2. *Qi* deficiency with insufficient body fluid type: Shortness of breath, general lassitude, dry mouth, constipation, sallow complexion, combined with palpitation, bad sleep, being woken up easily or dream-disturbed sleep, pale tongue and weak pulse.

Treatment Principle

Harmonizing the stomach and invigorating the spleen, removing obstruction and regulating *qi* activity.

Tuina Techniques

A. Gastric neurosis:

1. Pressing technique on the sternum.
2. Rubbing and pressing techniques on the upper abdomen.
3. Rubbing technique across the straight muscle of the abdomen.
4. Diagonal rubbing technique on the abdomen.
5. Straight rubbing technique on the lumbar region.

B. Intestinal neurosis:

1. Rubbing and pressing techniques on the upper abdomen.
2. Diagonal rubbing technique on the abdomen.
3. Rubbing and pressing techniques on the lower abdomen.
4. Rubbing technique on the back.

Addition or Subtraction Techniques

Gastric neurosis:

A. Spleen and stomach Yang deficiency type:

Addition: 1. Pressing technique on the upper abdomen. 2. Squeezing and pushing techniques on the back.

B. Liver and spleen Yin deficiency type:

Addition: 1. Pressing technique on the lower abdomen. 2. Squeezing and pushing techniques on the abdomen. 3. Digital pressing technique on the back.

Intestinal neurosis:

A. *Qi* obstruction with abdominal pain type:

Addition: 1. Diagonal rubbing technique on the hypochondriac region. 2. Digital pressing technique on the chest and abdomen. 3. Big relieving *qi* stagnation technique.

B. *Qi* deficiency with insufficient body fluid type:

Addition: 1. Holding and lifting techniques on the abdominal muscles. 2. Stationary circular pressing technique on Mingmen (GV 4).

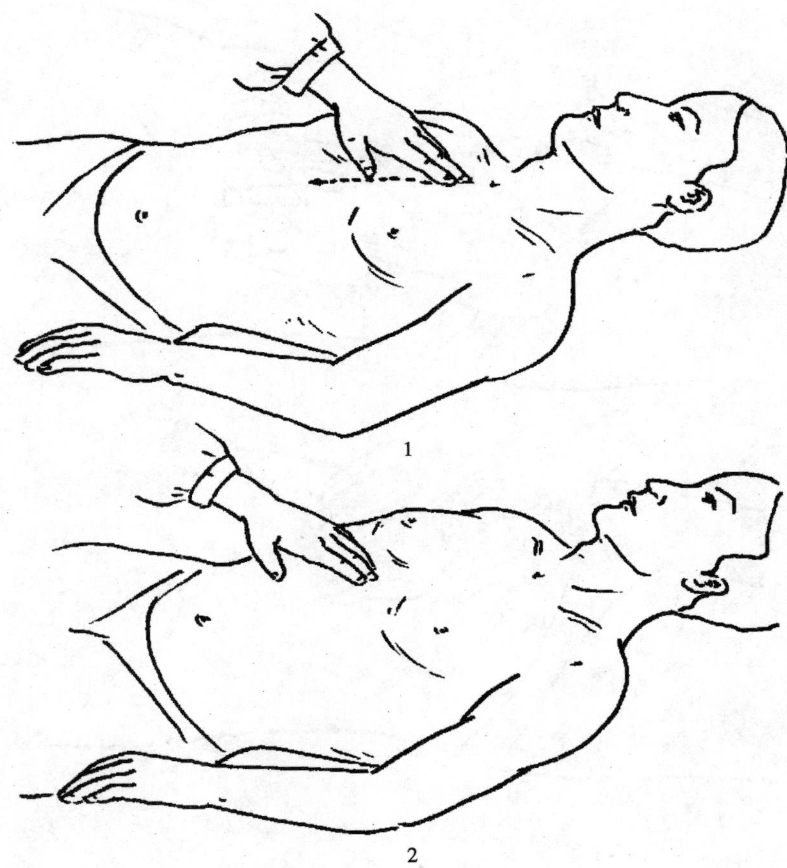

1

2

Pressing technique on the sternum.

Manipulation

Place four fingertips on Xuanji (CV 21), apply digital press method downwards along the anterior midline and stop at Zhongting (CV 16). Repeat the manipulation 2-3 minutes.

Points

1. Xuanji (CV 21): On the anterior midline, at the midpoint of the sternal angle, at the level with the first intercostal space.

2. Zhongting (CV 16): On the midline of the sternum, at the level with the fifth intercostal space.

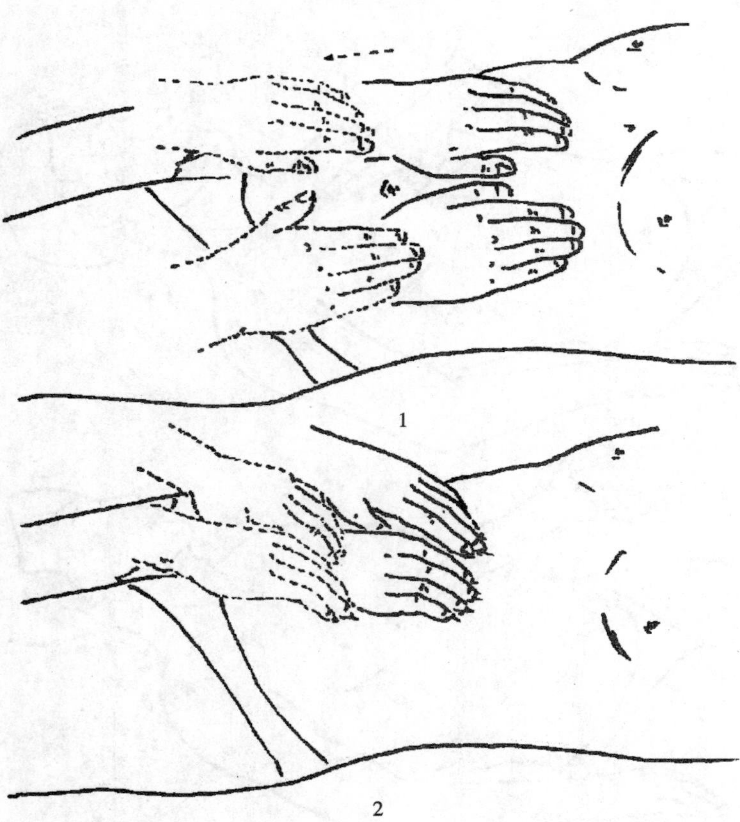

Rubbing and pressing techniques on the upper abdomen.

Manipulation

Place four finger-pulps of both hands on Burong (ST 19) and rub downwards to Tianshu (ST 25). Repeat the massage for 1-2 minutes, then press Burong (ST 19) and Tianshu (ST 25) for 1-2 minutes.

Points

1. Burong (ST 19): 6 *cun* above the umbilicus and 2 *cun* lateral to the midline.
2. Tianshu (ST 25): 2 *cun* lateral to the center of the umbilicus.

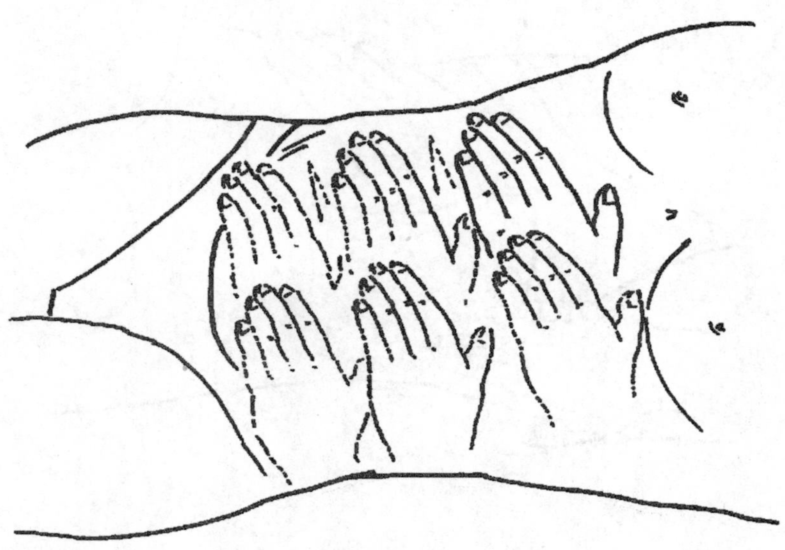

Rubbing technique across the straight muscle of the abdomen.

Manipulation

Place a palm on Youmen (KI 21), then rub the straight muscle of the abdomen transversely and stop at Henggu (KI 11). Repeat the manipulation 2-3 minutes.

Points

1. Youmen (KI 21): 6 *cun* above the center of the umbilicus and 0.5 *cun* lateral to the midline.

2. Henggu (KI 11): 5 *cun* below the center of the umbilicus and 0.5 *cun* lateral to the midline.

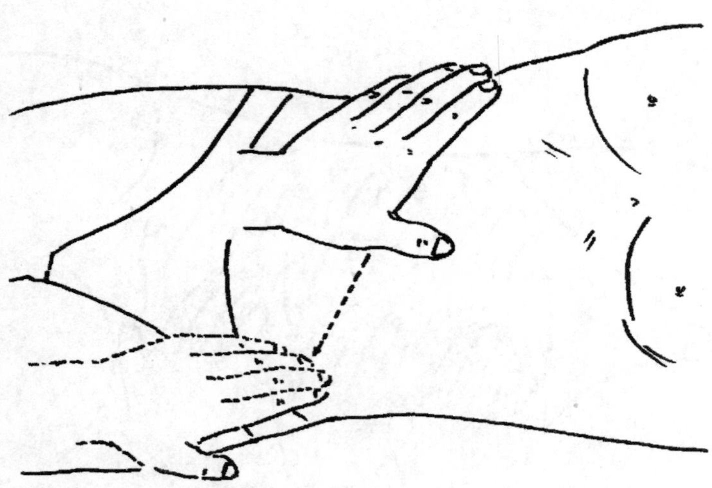

Diagonal rubbing technique on the abdomen.

Manipulation

Place a palm on one side of Fuai (SP 16), then rub diagonally downwards past Taiyi (ST 23), Shuifen (CV 9) and stop at the opposite Shuidao (ST 28) and Guilai (ST 29). Repeat the manipulation for 3-5 minutes.

Points

1. Fuai (SP 16): 3 *cun* above the center of the umbilicus and 4 *cun* lateral to the midline.
2. Taiyi (ST 23): 2 *cun* above the center of the umbilicus and 2 *cun* lateral to the midline.
3. Shuifen (CV 9): 1 *cun* above the center of the umbilicus.
4. Shuidao (ST 28): 3 *cun* below the center of the umbilicus and 2 *cun* lateral to the midline.
5. Guilai (ST 29): 4 *cun* below the center of the umbilicus and 2 *cun* lateral to the midline.

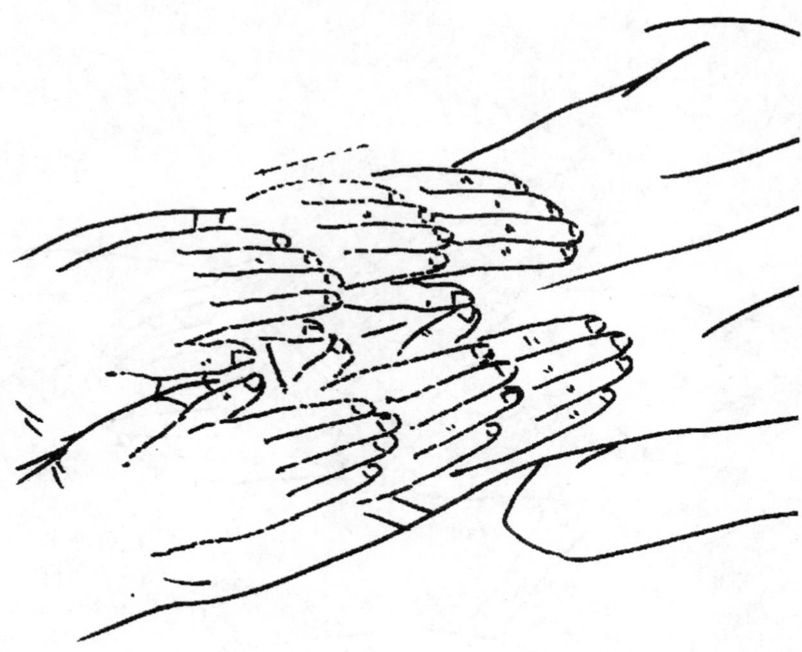

Straight rubbing technique on the lumbar region.

Manipulation

Place four finger-pulps of both hands on Weishu (BL 21) and Weicang (BL 50), rub straight downwards past Shenshu (BL 23), Zhishi (BL 52) and stop at Xiaochangshu (BL 27). Repeat the manipulation 5-15 minutes.

Points

1. Weishu (BL 21): At the level of the lower border of the spinous process of the twelfth thoracic vertebra and 1.5 *cun* lateral to the midline.

2. Weicang (BL 50): 1.5 *cun* lateral to Weishu (BL 21).

3. Shenshu (BL 23): At the level of the lower border of the spinous process of the second lumbar vertebra and 1.5 *cun* lateral to the midline.

4. Zhishi (BL 52): 1.5 *cun* lateral to Shenshu (BL 23).

5. Xiaochangshu (BL 27): At the level of the first posterior sacral foramen and 1.5 *cun* lateral to the midline.

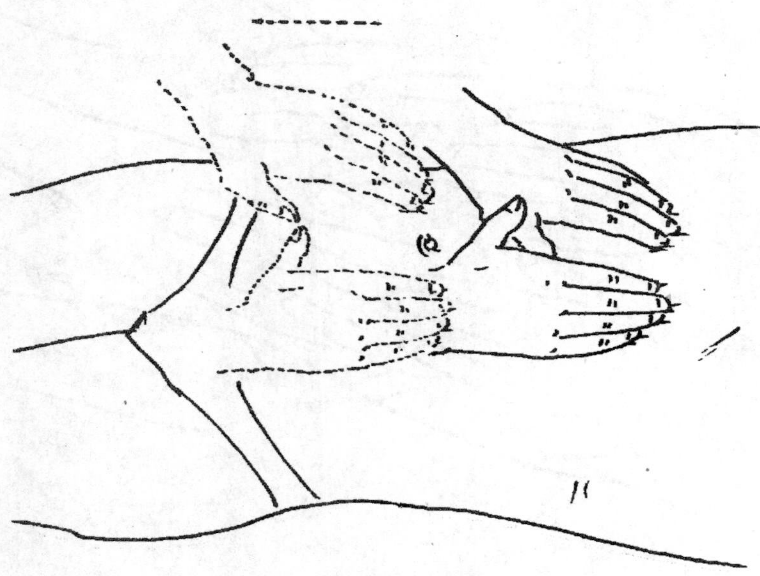

Pressing technique on the upper abdomen.

Manipulation

Place four fingertips of both hands on Youmen (KI 21), press and rub downwards to Huangshu (KI 16). Repeat the manipulation for 1-2 minutes.

Points

1. Youmen (KI 21): 6 *cun* above the center of the umbilicus and 0.5 *cun* lateral to the midline.

2. Huangshu (KI 16): 0.5 *cun* lateral to the center of the umbilicus.

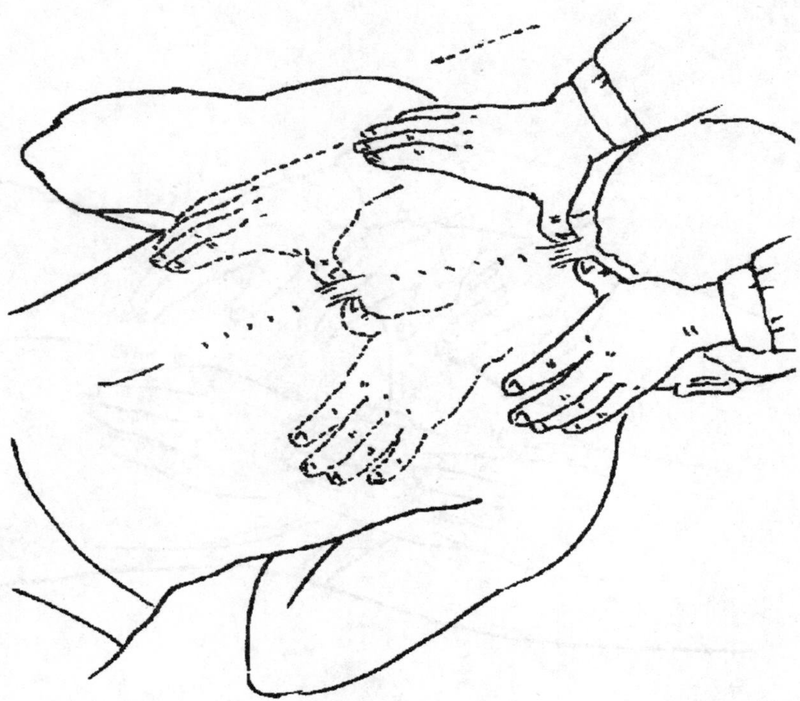

Squeezing and pushing techniques on the back.

Manipulation

With other fingers fanning out on each side of the back, place two thumb-pulps respectively on Dazhu (BL 11), then squeeze and push the back muscle slowly along the spine, and stop at Geshu (BL 17). Repeat the manipulation for 3-5 minutes.

Points

1. Dazhu (BL 11): At the level of the lower border of the spinous process of the first thoracic vertebra and 1.5 *cun* lateral to the midline.

2. Geshu (BL 17): At the level of the lower border of the spinous process of the seventh thoracic vertebra and 1.5 *cun* lateral to the midline.

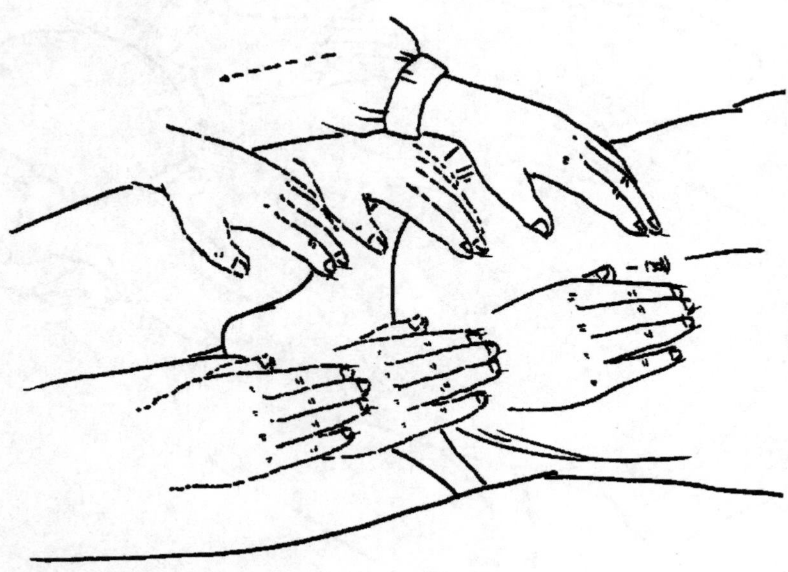

Pressing technique on the lower abdomen.

Manipulation

Place four finger-pulps of both hands on Huangshu (KI 16), then press and rub straight downwards to Siman (KI 14) and stop at Henggu (KI 11). Repeat the manipulation for 1-3 minutes.

Points

1. Huangshu (KI 16): 0.5 *cun* lateral to the center of the umbilicus.

2. Siman (KI 14): 2 *cun* below the center of the umbilicus and 0.5 *cun* lateral to the midline.

3. Henggu (KI 11): 5 *cun* below the center of the umbilicus and 0.5 *cun* lateral to the midline.

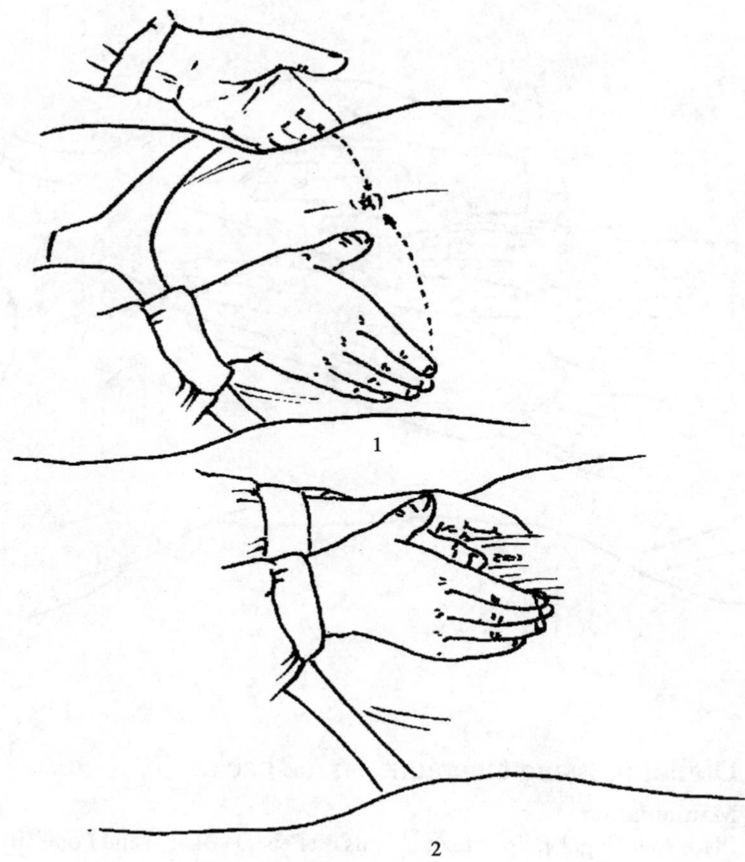
1

2

Squeezing and pushing techniques on the abdomen.

Manipulation

Place four finger-pulps of both hands on the two sides of Zhangmen (LR 13) and Jingmen (GB 25) of the abdomen, then squeeze and rub towards the middle of the abdomen. Repeat the manipulation for 2-3 minutes.

Points

1. Zhangmen (LR 13): On the lateral side of the abdomen, below the free end of the eleventh floating rib.

2. Jingmen (GB 25): On the lateral side of the abdomen, below the free end of the twelfth floating rib.

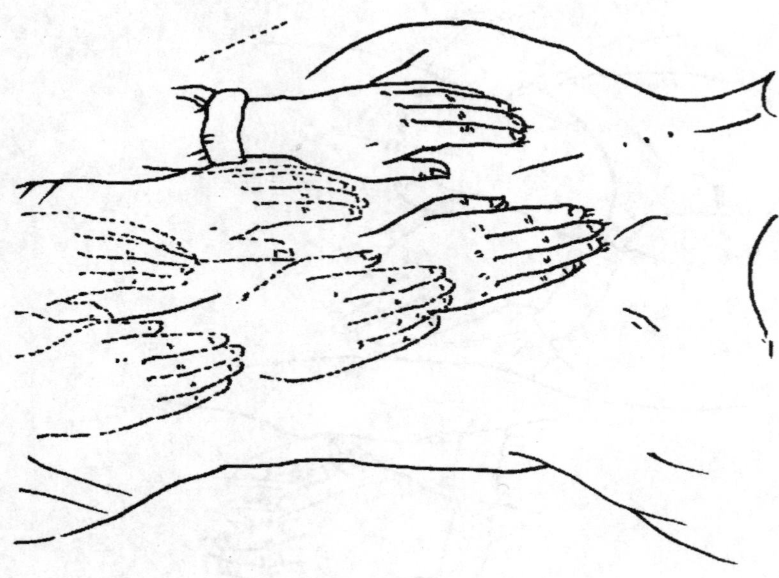

Digital pressing technique on the back.

Manipulation

Place four finger-pulps of both hands on Feishu (BL 13) and Pohu (BL 42), then slowly press the intercostal spaces in turn past Geshu (BL 17), Geguan (BL 46) and stop at Weishu (BL 21) and Weicang (BL 50). Repeat the manipulation for 3-5 times.

Points

1. Feishu (BL 13): At the level of the lower border of the spinous process of the third thoracic vertebra and 1.5 *cun* lateral to the midline.
2. Pohu (BL 42): 1.5 *cun* lateral to Feishu (BL 13).
3. Geshu (BL 17): At the level of the lower border of the spinous process of the seventh thoracic vertebra and 1.5 *cun* lateral to the midline.
4. Geguan (BL 46): 1.5 *cun* lateral to Geshu (BL 17).
5. Weishu (BL 21): At the level of the lower border of the spinous process of the twelfth thoracic vertebra and 1.5 *cun* lateral to the midline.
6. Weicang (BL 50): 1.5 *cun* lateral to Weishu (BL 21).

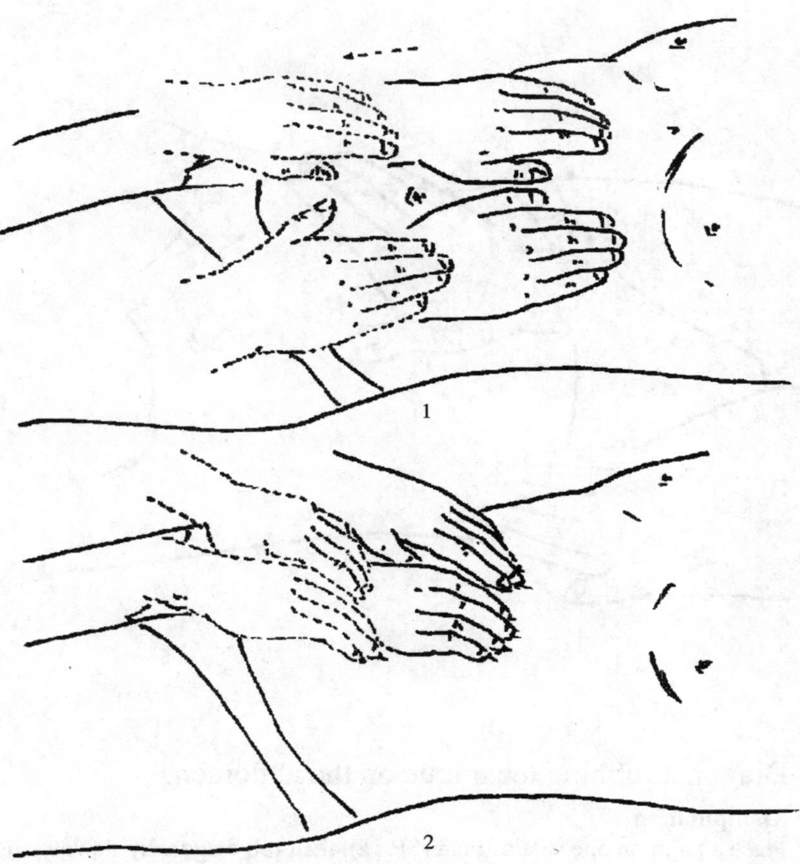

Rubbing and pressing techniques on the upper abdomen.

Manipulation

Place four finger-pulps of both hands on Burong (ST 19), then rub downwards to Tianshu (ST 25). Repeat the massage for 1-2 minutes, then apply point pressing on Burong (ST 19) and Tianshu (ST 25) for 1-2 minutes.

Points

1. Burong (ST 19): 6 *cun* above the umbilicus and 2 *cun* lateral to the midline.
2. Tianshu (ST 25): 2 *cun* lateral to the center of the umbilicus.

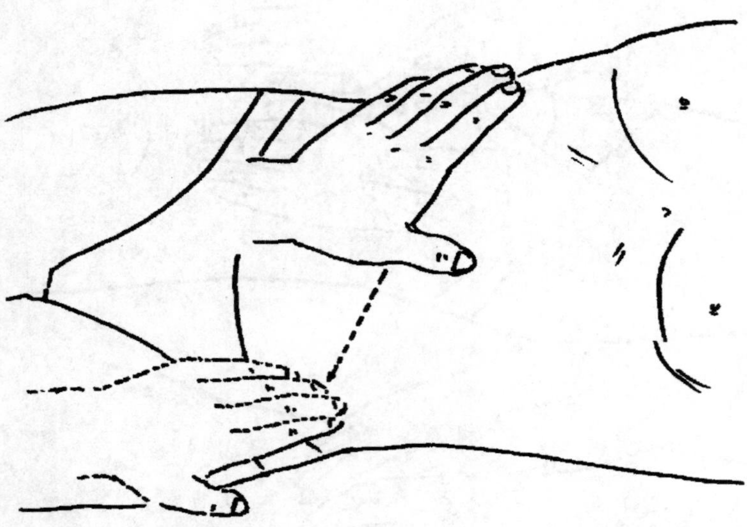

Diagonal rubbing technique on the abdomen.

Manipulation

Place a palm on one side of Fuai (SP 16), then rub diagonally downwards past Taiyi (ST 23), Shuifen (CV 9) and stop at the opposite Shuidao (ST 28) and Guilai (ST 29). Repeat the manipulation for 3-5 minutes.

Points

1. Fuai (SP 16): 3 *cun* above the center of the umbilicus and 4 *cun* lateral to the midline.

2. Taiyi (ST 23): 2 *cun* above the center of the umbilicus and 2 *cun* lateral to the midline.

3. Shuifen (CV 9): 1 *cun* above the center of the umbilicus and 2 *cun* lateral to the midline.

4. Shuidao (ST 28): 3 *cun* below the center of the umbilicus and 2 *cun* lateral to the midline.

5. Guilai (ST 29): 4 *cun* below the center of the umbilicus and 2 *cun* lateral to the midline.

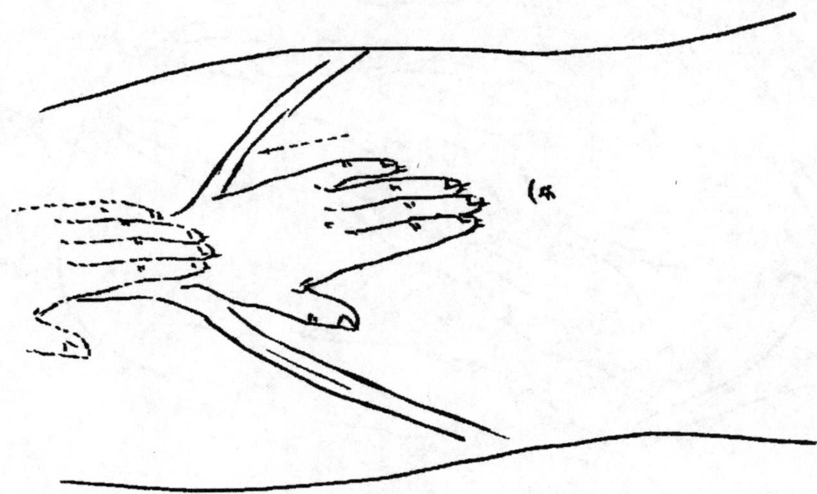

Rubbing and pressing techniques on the lower abdomen.

Manipulation

Place four finger-pulps of one hand on Yinjiao (CV 7), then press and rub straight downwards along the anterior midline to Qugu (CV 2). Repeat the manipulation for 1-2 minutes.

Points

1. Yinjiao (CV 7): 1 *cun* below the center of the umbilicus.
2. Qugu (CV 2): 5 *cun* below the center of the umbilicus.

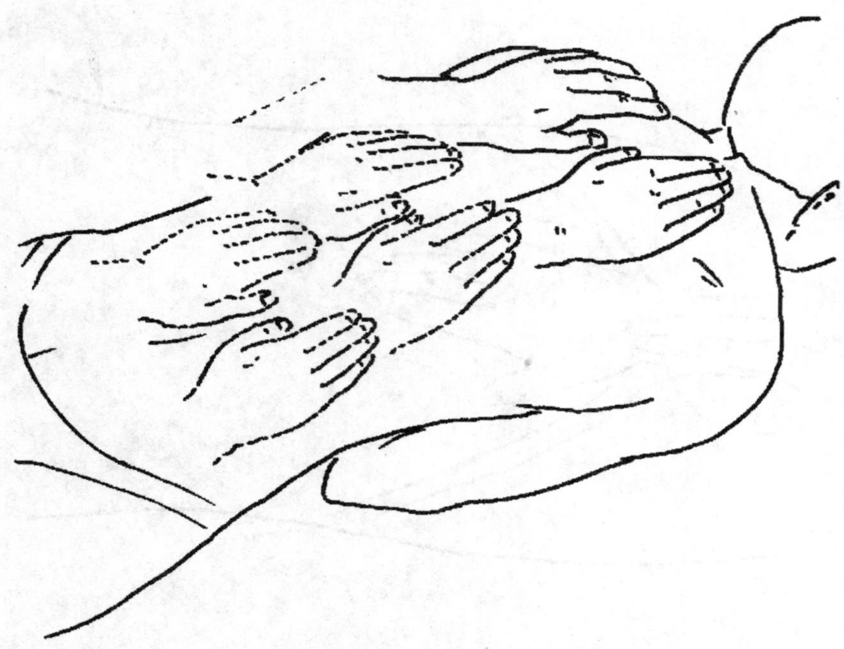

Rubbing technique on the back.

Manipulation

Place both palms flat on each side of the back, with both thumbs on Dazhui (GV 14), and slowly massage downwards along the spine past Zhiyang (GV 9) and stop at Xuanshu (GV 5), at the same time knead the points of the Governor Vessel with the thumbs. Repeat the manipulation for 3-5 minutes.

Points

1. Dazhui (GV 14): Below the spinous process of the seventh cervical vertebra.

2. Zhiyang (GV 9): Below the spinous process of the seventh thoracic vertebra.

3. Xuanshu (GV 5): Below the spinous process of the first lumbar vertebra.

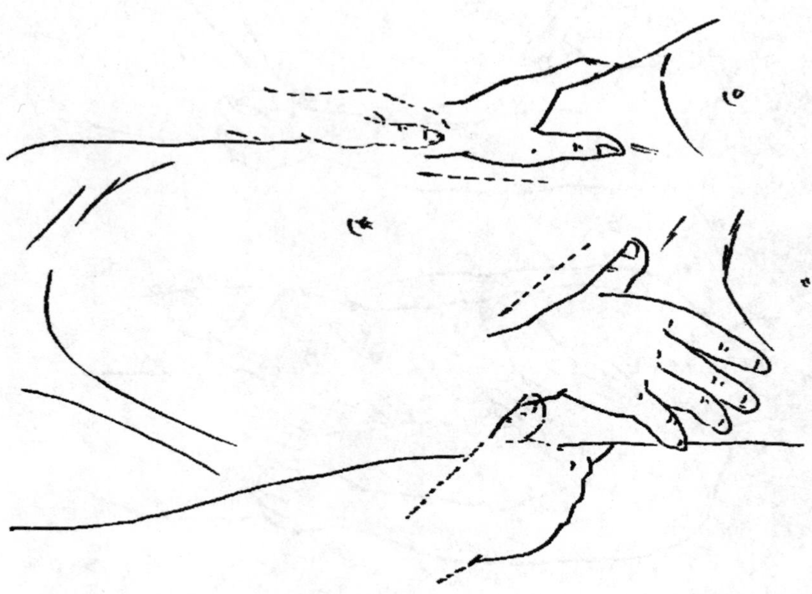

Diagonal rubbing technique on the hypochondrium.

Manipulation

Place two thumbs on Burong (ST 19) and Chengman (ST 20), then rub along the lower border of ribcage diagonally and stop at both sides of Zhangmen (LR 13). Repeat the manipulation for 3-5 minutes.

Points

1. Burong (ST 19): 6 *cun* above the center of the umbilicus and 2 *cun* lateral to the midline.

2. Chengman (ST 20): 5 *cun* above the center of the umbilicus and 2 *cun* lateral to the midline.

3. Zhangmen (LR 13): On the lateral side of the abdomen, below the free end of the eleventh floating rib.

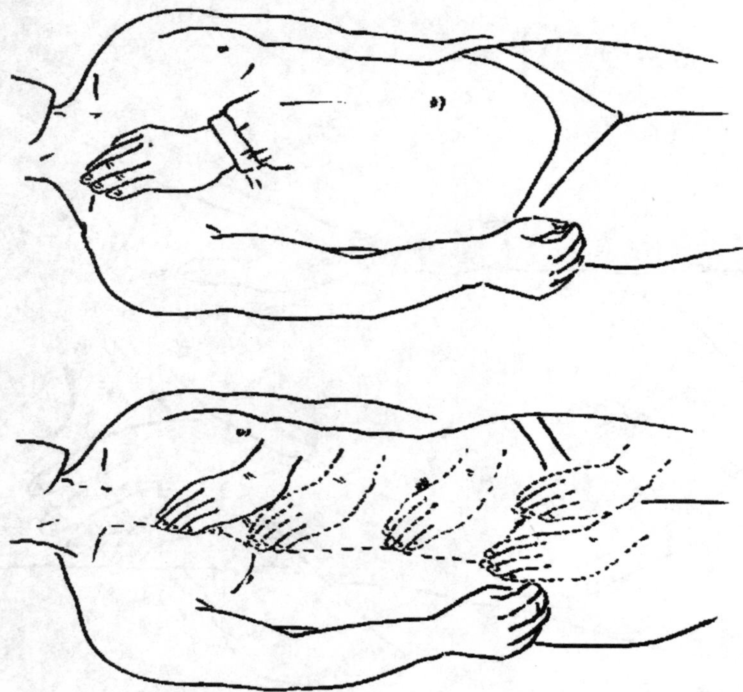

Digital pressing technique on chest and abdomen.

Manipulation

Place four fingertips of one hand on Qihu (ST 13), then slowly press the intercostal space downwards along Yingchuang (ST 16), Qimen (LR 14), Daheng (SP 15), Fushe (SP 13), and stop at Qichong (ST 30). Repeat the manipulation 2-3 times.

Points

1. Qihu (ST 13): At the lower border of the middle of the clavicle, 4 *cun* lateral to the anterior midline.
2. Yingchuang (ST 16): In the third intercostal space, 4 *cun* lateral to the anterior midline.
3. Qimen (LR 14): Directly below the nipple, in the sixth intercostal space.
4. Daheng (SP 15): 4 *cun* lateral to the center of the umbilicus.
5. Fushe (SP 13): 3.5 *cun* below the center of the umbilicus and 4 *cun* lateral to the anterior midline.
6. Qichong (ST 30): 5 *cun* below the center of the umbilicus and 2 *cun* lateral to the anterior midline.

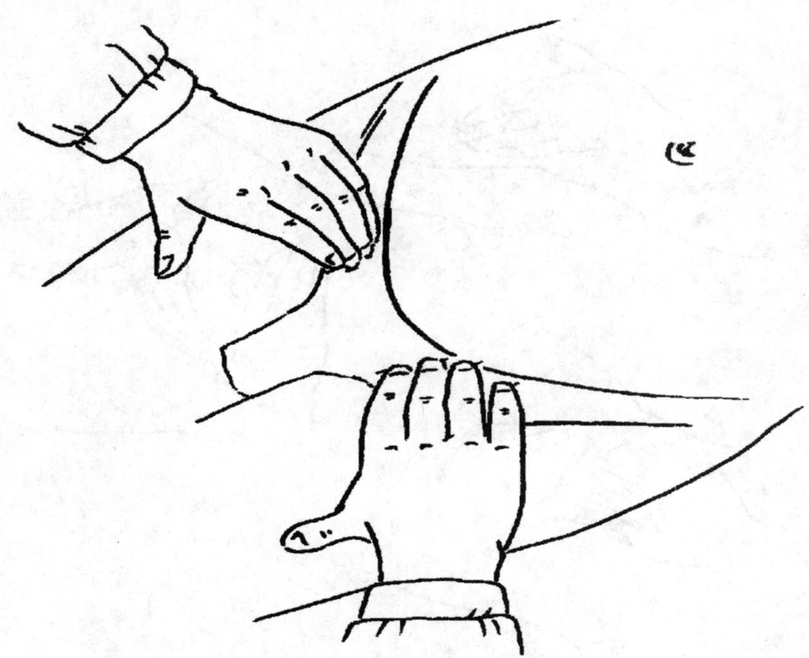

Big relieving *qi* stagnation technique.

Manipulation

Place four finger-pulps of both hands on bilateral Guilai (ST 29) and Qichong (ST 30) located at the lower abdomen. Press the points 1-3 times, each time should last 15-60 seconds.

Points

1. Guilai (ST 29): 4 *cun* below the center of the umbilicus and 2 *cun* lateral to the midline.

2. Qichong (ST 30): 5 *cun* below the center of the umbilicus and 2 *cun* lateral to the midline.

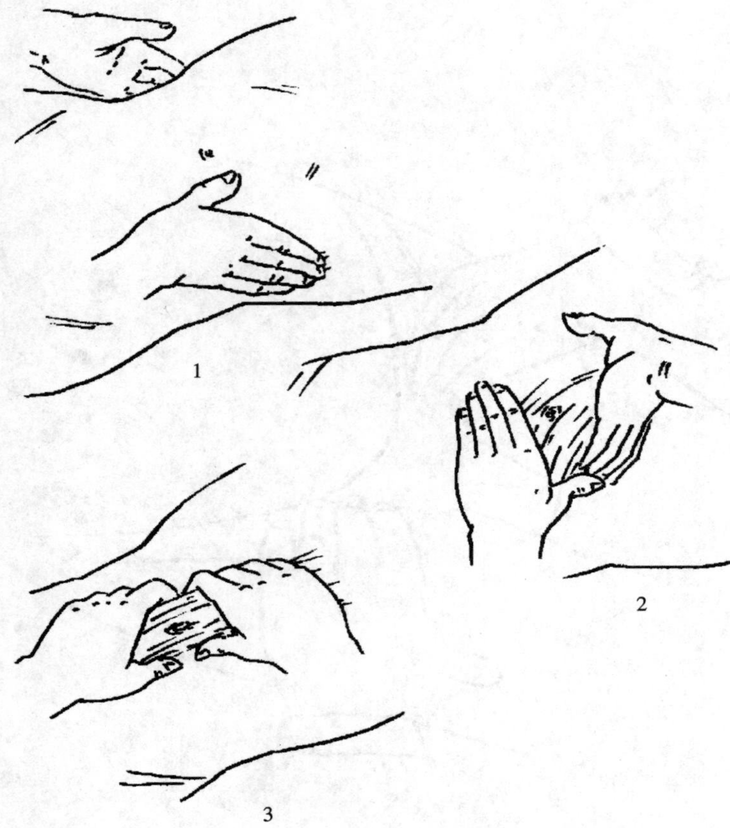

Holding and lifting techniques on the abdominal muscles.

Manipulation

Place respectively the four finger-pulps of both hands on bilateral Zhangmen (LR 13), squeeze and push vigorously the abdominal muscles towards the middle of the abdomen. Turn one hand while the other hand keeps pushing the muscle, then with both hands grasp and lift the squeezed abdominal muscle at the middle of the abdomen 3-5 times. Each time lasts 5-10 seconds.

Points

Zhangmen (LR 13): On the lateral side of the abdomen, below the free end of the eleventh floating rib.

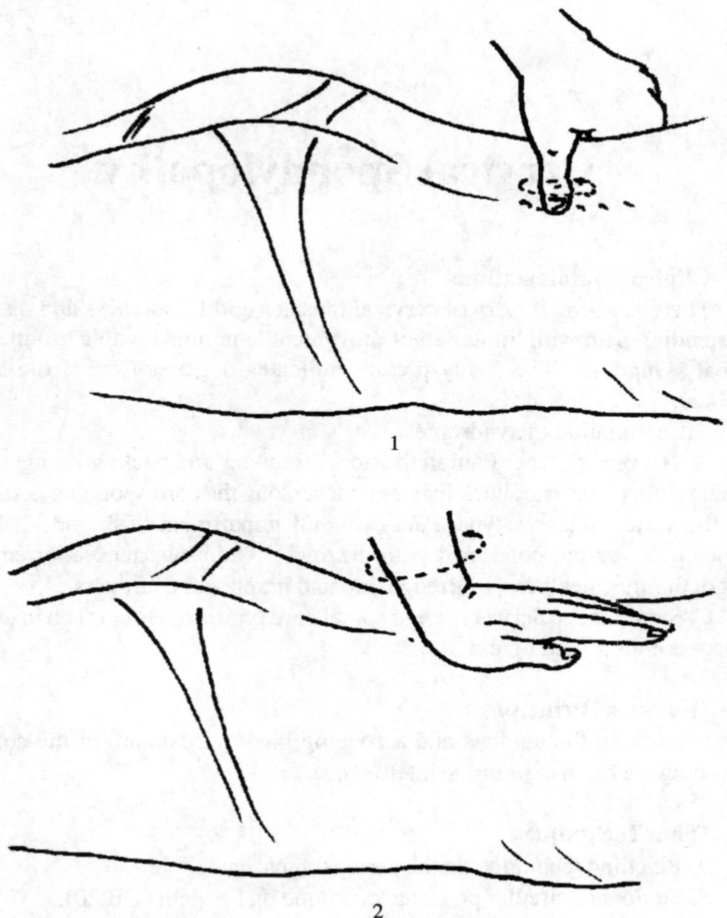

1

2

Stationary circular pressing technique on Mingmen (GV 4).

Manipulation

Place a thumb on Mingmen (GV 4) and knead the point for 2-3 minutes, then place the palm flat on the same area and conduct circular pressing with the palm for 1-2 minutes.

Points

Mingmen (GV 4): Below the spinous process of the second lumbar vertebra.

Cervical Spondylopathy

Clinical Manifestations

There is a long history of cervical muscle rigidity, soreness and distention, or distending pain with limitation of movement, combined with a group of other clinical symptoms. The X-ray picture indicates degeneration of the cervical vertebrae.

Differentiation of syndromes:

A. Nerve root type: Pain in the neck, shoulder and back; burning or sharp, stabbing pain, or electric shock like numbness along the corresponding dermatome.

B. Vertebral artery type: Pain or motor impairment of the neck, shoulder and occipital region; combined with dizziness, vomiting, nausea, orientational vertigo, tinnitus, deafness, blurred vision and numbness of fingers.

C. Sympathetic nerve type and spinal cord type are seldom seen in clinic, so they are not discussed herein.

Treatment Principle

Smoothing the tendons and activating blood circulation in the collateral, reinforcing the brain to improve intelligence.

Tuina Techniques

A. Pinching technique on the cervical muscles.

B. Stationary circular pressing technique on Fengchi (GB 20).

C. Separate pushing technique on the occipital region.

D. Pressing technique on Wangu (GB 12).

E. Holding technique on Jianjing (GB 21).

F. Neck rotation while pressing the shoulder technique.

Addition or Subtraction Techniques

A. Nerve root type:

Addition: 1. Pushing and pressing techniques on the three points of Yangming meridians. 2. Pressing technique on Jiquan (HT 1). 3. Pressing technique on Quepen (ST 12).

B. Vertebral artery type:

Addition: 1. Separate pushing technique on the forehead. 2. Stationary circular pressing technique on Taiyang (Ex-HN 5). 3. Opposite pressing technique on the head. 4. Pushing technique along the Governor Vessel on the head. 5. Opposite pressing technique on Waiguan (TE 5) and Neiguan (PC 6).

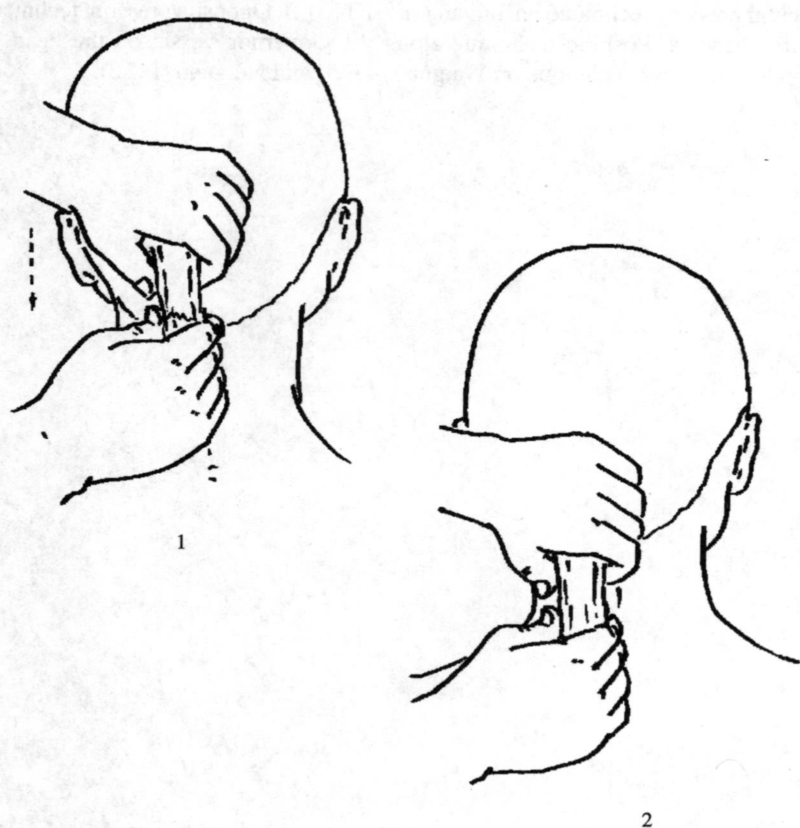

1

2

Pinching technique on the cervical muscles.

Manipulation

Use fingers of both hands to pinch and pull up the neck muscle on the side of the neck starting from Fengchi (GB 20) down to Jianzhongshu (SI 15). Repeat the manipulation for 1-2 minutes on each side of the neck.

Points

1. Fengchi (GB 20): In the depression between the upper portion of m. sternocleidomastoideus and m. trapezius, on the same level with Fengfu (GV 16).

2. Jianzhongshu (SI 15): 2 *cun* lateral to the lower border of the spinous process of the seventh cervical vertebra.

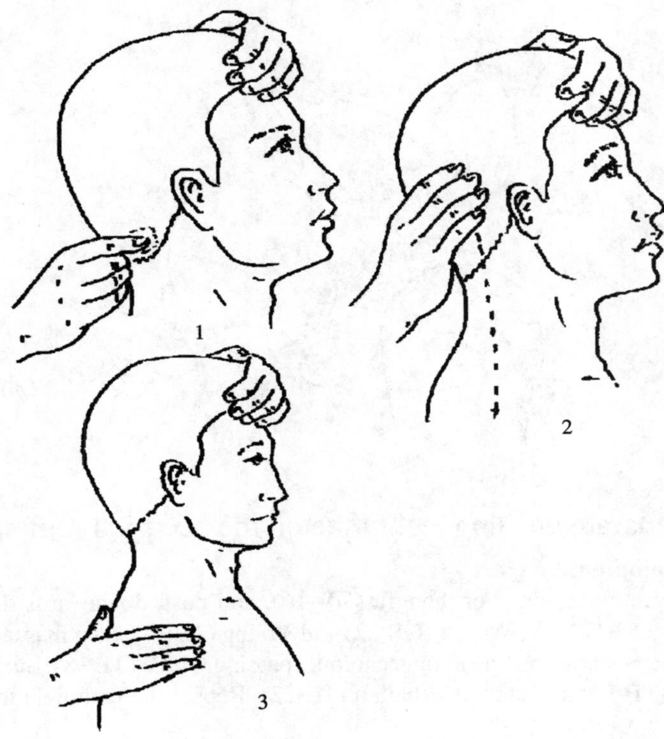

Stationary circular pressing technique on Fengchi (GB 20).

Manipulation

1. Place one hand on the front of forehead to keep it still as the thumb and index finger of the other hand knead Fengchi (GB 20) for 1-3 minutes.

2. Place four finger-pulps of one hand at Naokong (GB 19), then push and rub downwards past Fengchi (GB 20) and stop at Jianjing (GB 21), (See figures 2 and 3). Treat both sides, repeat the massage at each side for 1-3 minutes.

Points

1. Fengchi (GB 20): In the depression between the upper portion of m. sternocleidomastoideus and m. trapezius, on the same level with Fengfu (GV 16).

2. Naokong (GB 19): 1.5 *cun* above Fengchi (GB 20).

3. Jianjing (GB 21): Midway between the lower border of the spinous process of the seventh cervical vertebra and the acromion.

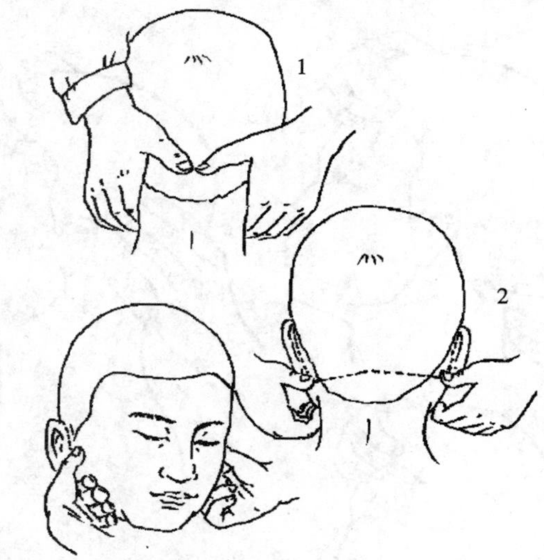

Separate pushing technique on the occipital region.

Manipulation

Place two thumbs on Fengfu (GV 16), and push downwards diagonally, past Fengchi (GB 20), Wangu (GB 12) and Yifeng (TE 17), then massage behind the ears in pushing and kneading technique, passing Qimai (TE 18), Luxi (TE 19), Jiaosun (TE 20) and stop at Erheliao (TE 22). Repeat the manipulation for 2-3 minutes.

Points

1. Fengfu (GV 16):1 *cun* directly above the midpoint of the posterior hairline.
2. Fengchi (GB 20): In the depression between the upper portion of m. Sternocleidomastoideus and m. trapezius, on the same level with Fengfu (GV 16).
3. Wangu (GB 12): In the depression posterior and inferior to the mastoid process.
4. Yifeng (TE 17): Posterior to the lobule of the ear, in the depression between the mandible and mastoid process.
5. Qimai (TE 18): In the center of the mastoid process, at the junction of the middle and lower third of the curve formed by Yifeng (TE 17) and Jiaosun (TE 20) posterior to the helix.
6. Luxi (TE 19): Posterior to the ear, at the junction of the upper and middle third of the curve formed by Yifeng (TE 17) and Jiaosun (TE 20) behind the helix.
7. Jiaosun (TE 20): Directly above the ear apex, within the hair-line.
8. Erheliao (TE 22): Anterior and superior to Ermen (TE 21), at the level with the root of the auricle, on the posterior border of the hairline of the temple where the superficial temporal artery passes.

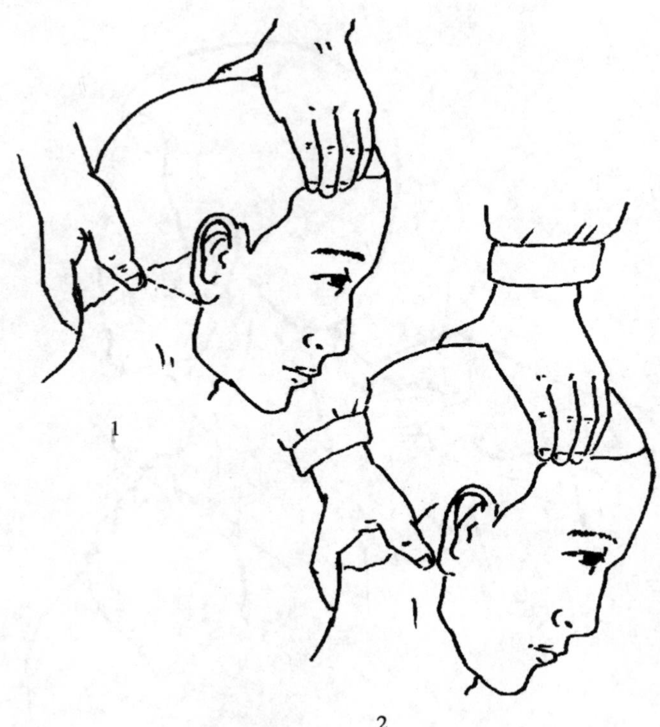

Pressing technique on Wangu (GB 12).

Manipulation

Place one thumb on Wangu (GB 12) and massage in kneading method for 1-2 minutes, then push to Yifeng (TE 17). Repeat the manipulation 1-2 minutes.

Points

1. Wangu (GB 12): In the depression posterior and inferior to the mastoid process.

2. Yifeng (TE 17): Posterior to the lobule of the ear, in the depression between the mandible and mastoid process.

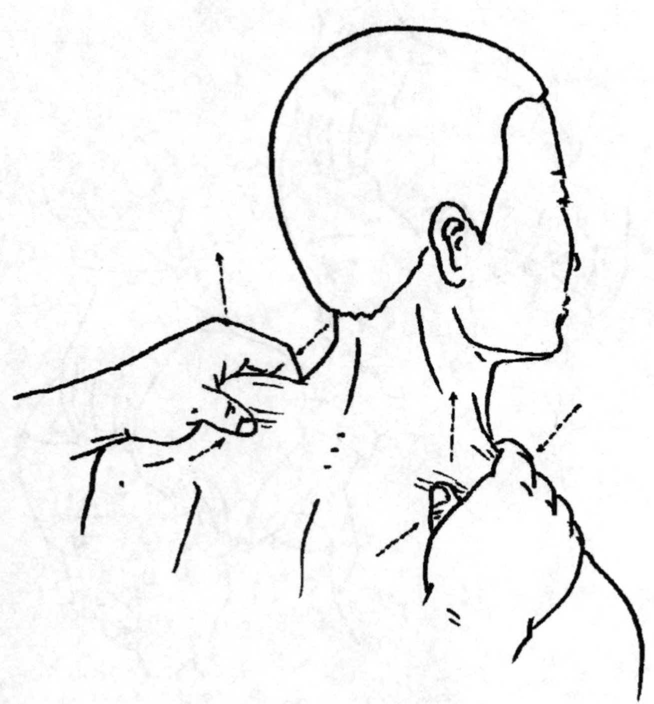

Holding technique on Jianjing (GB 21).

Manipulation

Place two thumbs respectively below Jianjing (GB 21) and other fingers at the front of the shoulder. Then grasp and lift the shoulder muscles with wrist strength 3-5 times, each time should last 10-20 seconds.

Points

Jianjing (GB 21): Midway between the lower border of the spinous process of the seventh cervical vertebra and the acromion.

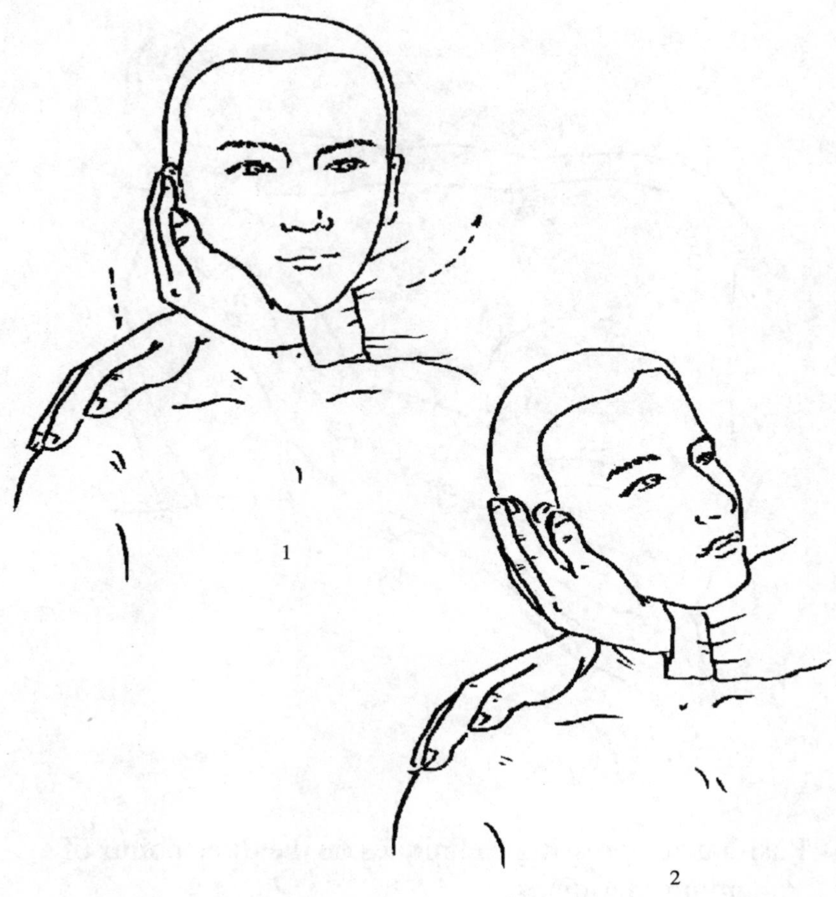

Neck rotation while pressing the shoulder technique.

Manipulation

Place one palm, which passes the nape, on the shoulder. Let the other hand go through the front of head to hold steadily the head, then turn the neck towards one side and slightly pull it in an outward and upward direction. Repeat the manipulation for 1-2 minutes.

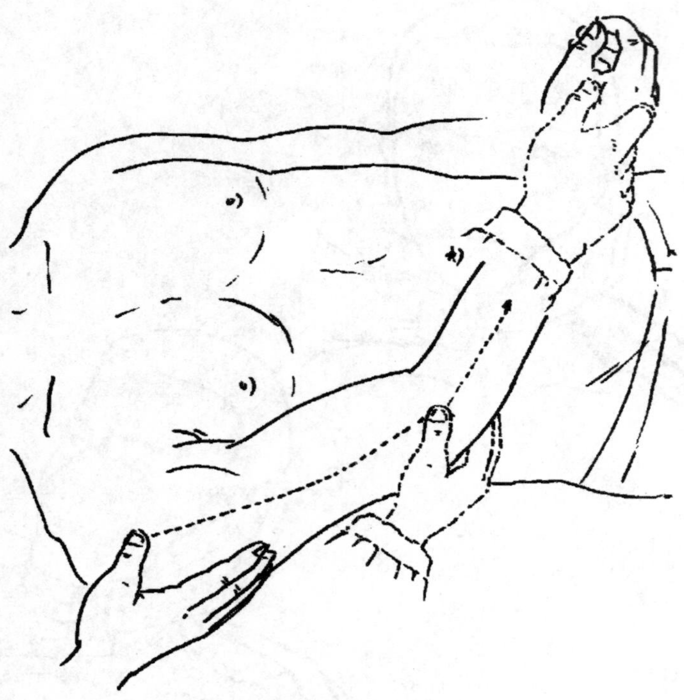

Pushing and pressing techniques on the three points of Yangming Meridians.

Manipulation

Place a thumb on Jianyu (LI 15), then push downwards along the arm, past Quchi (LI 11) and stop at Hegu (LI 4). Repeat the manipulation for 1-3 minutes.

Points

1. Jianyu (LI 15): In the depression appearing at the anterior border of the acromioclavicular joint when the arm is in full abduction.

2. Quchi (LI 11): In the depression at the lateral end of the transverse cubital crease.

3. Hegu (LI 4): On the dorsum of the hand, between the first and second metacarpal bones, approximately in the middle of the second metacarpal bone on the radial side.

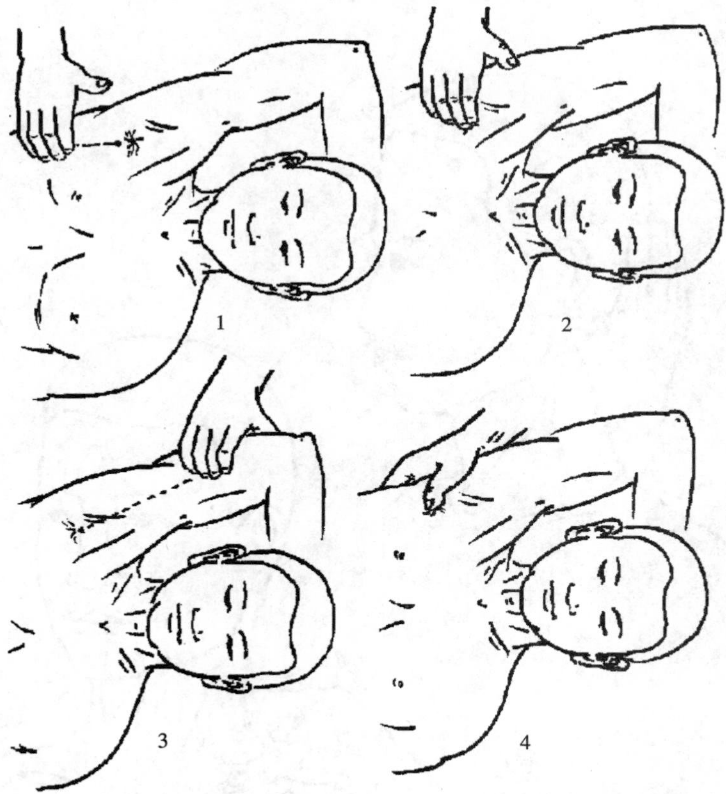

Pressing technique on Jiquan (HT 1).

Manipulation

Place four fingers on Yuanye (GB 22), and rub upwards to Jiquan (HT 1), then place fingers on Qingling (HT 2) and rub to Jiquan (HT 1). Repeat each manipulation for 1-2 minutes. Then place the thumb on Jiquan (HT 1) while wrapping with other fingers around the back of the shoulder. Press Jiquan (HT 1) with the thumb 2-3 times, each time should last 30-60 seconds.

Points

1. Yuanye (GB 22): On the mid-axillary line, in the fourth intercostal space.

2. Qingling (HT 2): 3 *cun* directly above the medial end of the transverse cubital crease.

3. Jiquan (HT 1): In the center of the axilla, on the medial side of the axillary artery.

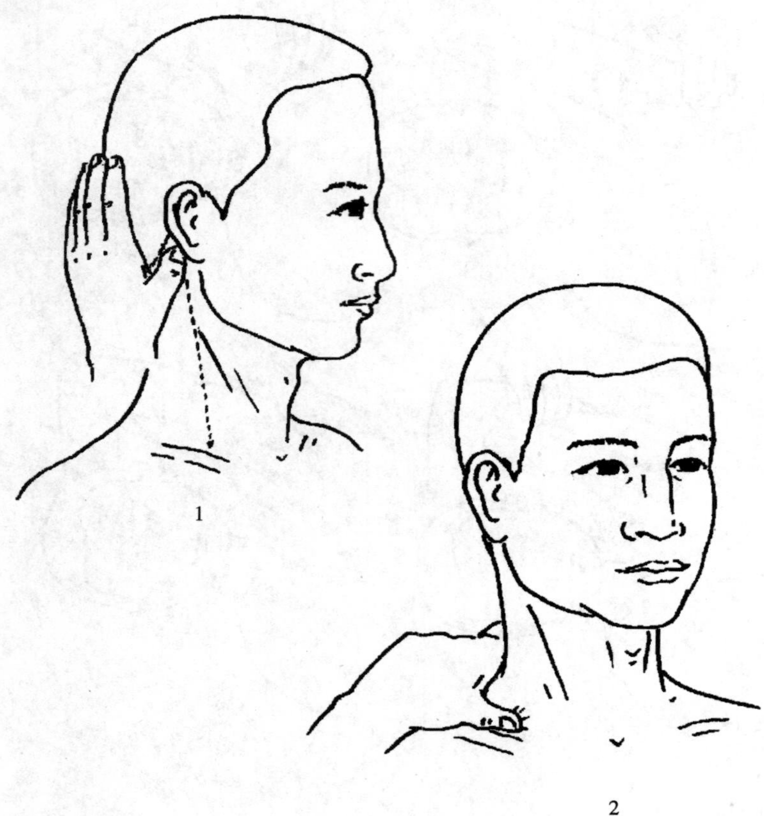

1

2

Pressing technique on Quepen (ST 12).

Manipulation

Place a thumb on Yifeng (TE 17), and apply massage down the neck in rubbing technique along the sternocleidomastoid muscle to Quepen (ST 12). Perform the manipulation 5-10 times. Then press Quepen (ST 12) 2-3 times, each time should last 15-30 seconds.

Points

1. Yifeng (TE 17): Posterior to the lobule of the ear, in the depression between the mandible and mastoid process.

2. Quepen (ST 12): In the midpoint of the supraclavicular fossa, 4 *cun* lateral to the anterior midline.

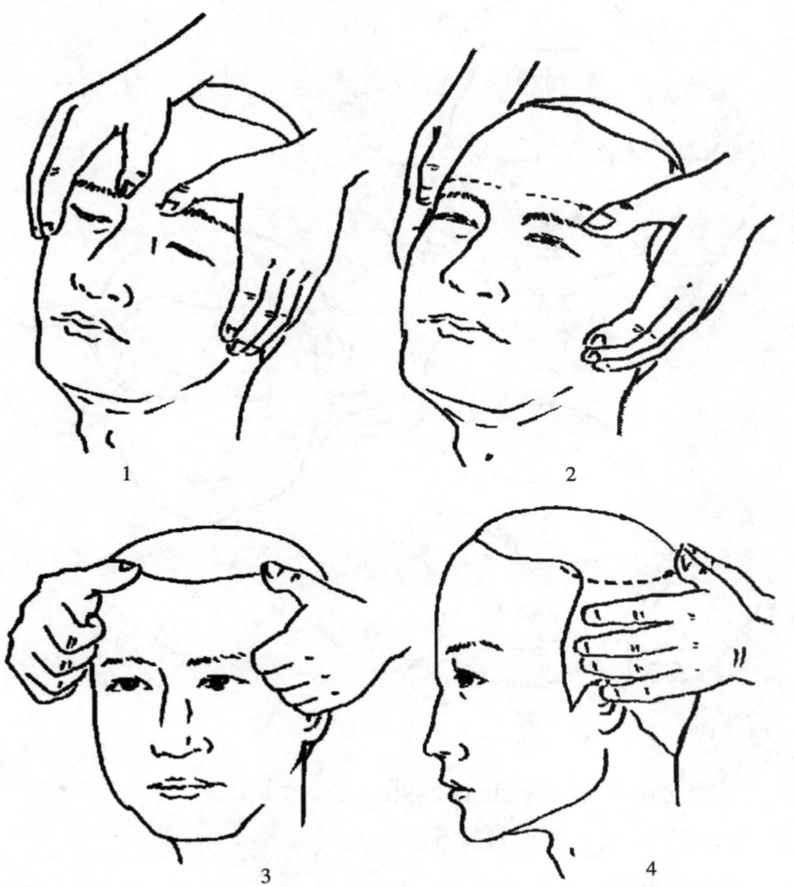

Separate pushing technique on the forehead.

Manipulation

Place two thumbs on the forehead center, then apply the massage with the thumbs pushing respectively to the sides of the forehead for 1-3 minutes. Then place two thumbs respectively on Touwei (ST 8), and rub backward to Houding (GV 19). Repeat the massage 1-2 minutes.

Points

1. Touwei (ST 8): 0.5 *cun* within the anterior hairline at the corner of the forehead, 4.5 *cun* lateral to the midline.

2. Houding (GV 19): On the midline of the head, 5.5 *cun* directly above the posterior hairline.

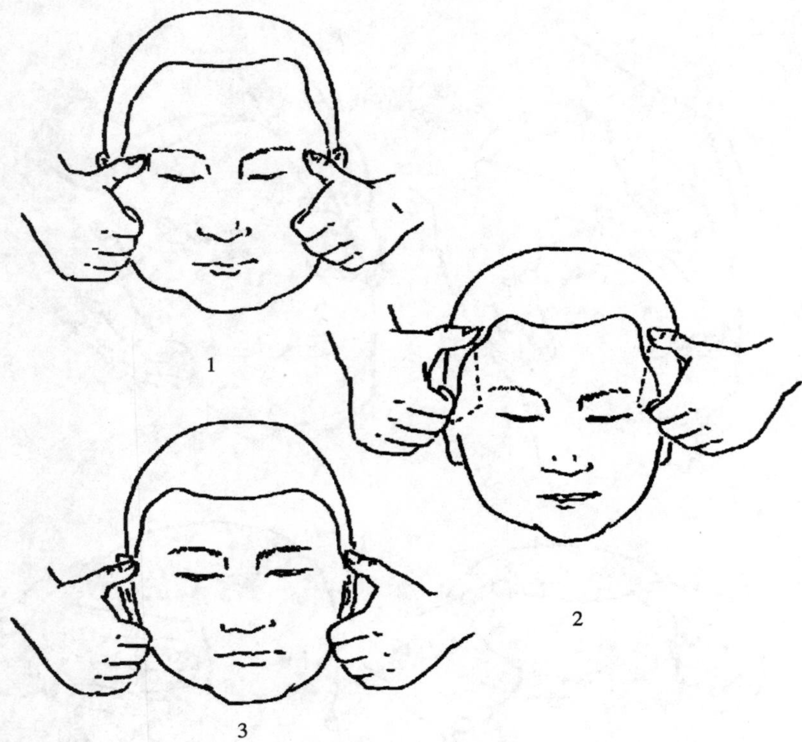

Stationary circular pressing technique on Taiyang (Ex-HN 5).

Manipulation

1. Place two thumbs respectively on bilateral Taiyang (Ex-HN 5) and knead for 1-3 minutes.

2. Move the thumbs from Taiyang (Ex-HN 5) to Touwei (ST 8), push and rub down to Taiyang (Ex-HN 5) then to Ermen (TE 21). Repeat the massage for 2-5 minutes.

Points

1. Taiyang (Ex-HN 5): In the depression about 1 *cun* posterior to the midpoint between the lateral end of the eyebrow and the outer canthus.

2. Touwei (ST 8): 0.5 *cun* within the anterior hairline at the corner of the forehead, 4.5 *cun* lateral to the midline.

3. Ermen (TE 21): In the depression anterior to the supratragic notch and slightly superior to the condyloid process of the mandible.

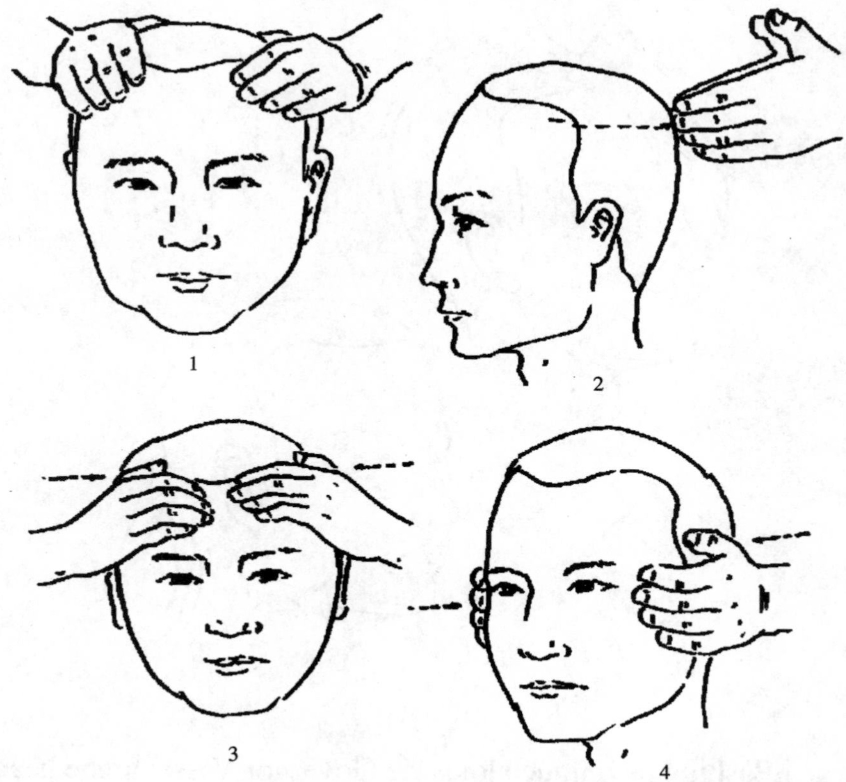

Opposite pressing technique on the head.

Manipulation

1. Place four finger-pulps of each hand on Touwei (ST 8) located at the side of the forehead, massage backward to Houding (GV 19) in rubbing technique, repeat it 1-3 minutes.

2. Let the palms press the temple regions vigorously, then the ears for 1-3 minutes.

Points

1. Touwei (ST 8): 0.5 *cun* within the anterior hairline at the corner of the forehead, 4.5 *cun* lateral to the midline.

2. Houding (GV 19): On the midline of the head, 5.5 *cun* directly above the posterior hairline.

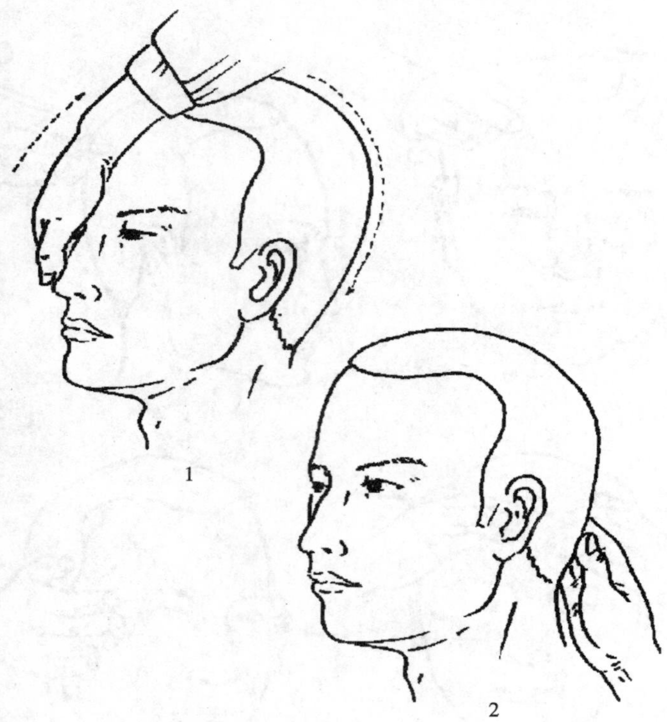

Pushing technique along the Governor Vessel at the head.

Manipulation

Place one thumb on Suliao (GV 25), rub straight upward, then downward along the Governor Vessel past Yintang (Ex-HN 3), Shenting (GV 24), Baihui (GV 20), Qiangjian (GV 18), and stop at Yamen (GV 15). Repeat the manipulation for 1-2 minutes.

Points

1. Suliao (GV 25): On the tip of the nose.
2. Yintang (Ex-HN 3): Midway between the medial ends of the two eyebrows.
3. Shenting (GV 24): 0.5 *cun* directly above the midpoint of the anterior hairline.
4. Baihui (GV 20): 7 *cun* directly above the midpoint of the posterior hairline.
5. Qiangjian (GV 18): 4 *cun* directly above the midpoint of the posterior hairline.
6. Yamen (GV 15): 0.5 *cun* directly above the midpoint of the posterior hairline.

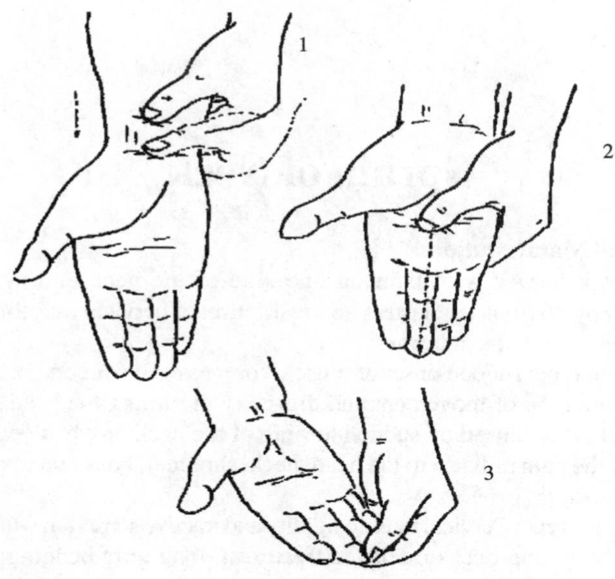

Opposite pressing technique on Waiguan (TE 5) and Neiguan (PC 6).

Manipulation

Place one thumb tip on Neiguan (PC 6) and other four fingertips on Waiguan (TE 5). Press the two acupoints for 1-2 minutes, then press and push downwards past Daling (PC 7) and Yangchi (TE 4) to Laogong (PC 8) and Zhongchong (PC 9). Rub each acupoint for 1-2 minutes. Repeat the manipulation for 1-3 times.

Points

1. Neiguan (PC 6): 2 *cun* above the transverse crease of the wrist, between the tendons of m. palmaris longus and m. flexor radialis.

2. Waiguan (TE 5): 2 *cun* above the transverse crease of the dorsum of wrist, between the radius and ulna.

3. Daling (PC 7): In the middle of the transverse crease of the wrist, between the tendons of m. palmaris longus and m. flexor carpi radialis.

4. Yangchi (TE 4): On the transverse crease of the dorsum of wrist, in the depression lateral to the tendon of m. extensor digitorum communis.

5. Laogong (PC 8): On the transverse crease of the palm, between the second and third metacarpal bones.

6. Zhongchong (PC 9): In the center of the tip of the middle finger.

Sprain of Neck

Clinical Manifestations

The neck is wry with pain on one side of the neck and upper back, accompanied by obvious tenderness and restriction of cervical mobility.

Differentiation of syndromes:

A. Acute type: sudden onset of muscle soreness and pain on one side of the neck, with limitation of movement and difficulty in turning the head to the left, right and back. It is caused by sudden turning of the neck or when getting up. In severe cases, the pain radiates to the head, neck, shoulder, back and upper limb of the affected side.

B. Chronic type: Cervical muscle rigidity and tractive sensation while moving, caused mainly by improper or delayed treatment, long term bending of head at work, or overstrain of the cervical muscles; these symptoms are relieved temporarily after massage and usually occur bilaterally with the manifestations of compensatory cervical muscle strain, often combined with dizziness, headache, insomnia, etc. This type of sprain may induce cervical spondylosis or become one of its causative factors.

Treatment Principle

Smoothing the tendon, activating blood circulation in the collateral and relieving the pain.

Tuina Techniques

A. Pinching technique on the cervical muscle.

B. Separate pushing technique on the occipital region.

C. Holding technique on Jianjing (GB 21).

D. Kneading technique on Hegu (LI 4).

Addition or Subtraction Techniques

A. Acute type:

Addition: 1. Stationary circular pressing technique on Fengchi (GB 20). 2. Neck rotation technique.

B. Chronic type:

Addition: 1. Finger stationary circular pressing technique on Quyuan (SI 13). 2. Neck rotation while pressing the shoulder technique.

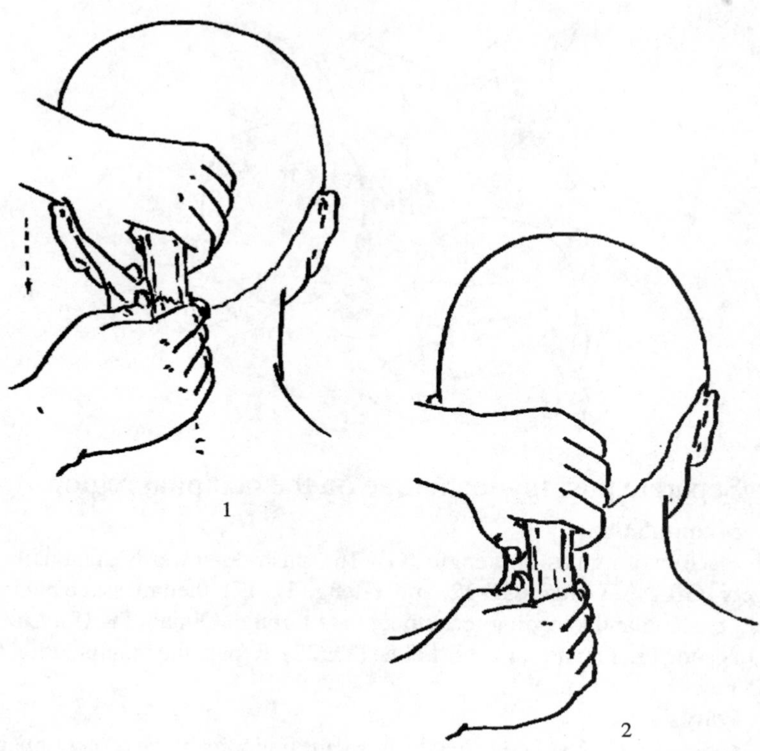

Pinching technique on the cervical muscles.

Manipulation

Use fingers of both hands to pinch and pull up the neck muscle on the side of the neck starting from Fengchi (GB 20) down to Jianzhongshu (SI 15). Repeat the manipulation for 1-2 minutes on each side of the neck.

Points

1. Fengchi (GB 20): In the depression between the upper portion of m. sternocleidomastoideus and m. trapezius, on the same level with Fengfu (GV 16).

2. Jianzhongshu (SI 15): 2 *cun* lateral to the lower border of the spinous process of the seventh cervical vertebra.

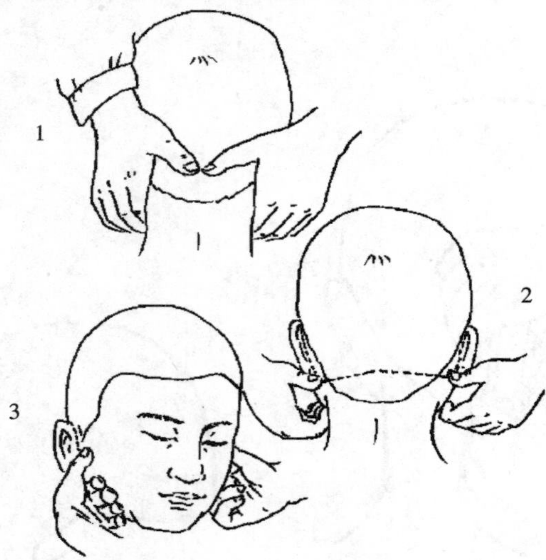

Separate pushing technique on the occipital region.

Manipulation

Place two thumbs on Fengfu (GV 16), push downwards diagonally, past Fengchi (GB 20), Wangu (GB 12) and Yifeng (TE 17), then massage behind the ears in pushing and kneading technique, pass through Qimai (TE 18), Luxi (TE 19), Jiaosun (TE 20) and stop at Erheliao (TE 22). Repeat the manipulation for 2-3 minutes.

Points

1. Fengfu (GV16):1 *cun* directly above the midpoint of the posterior hairline.
2. Fengchi (GB 20): In the depression between the upper portion of m. Sternocleidomastoideus and m. trapezius, on the same level with Fengfu (GV 16).
3. Wangu (GB 12): In the depression posterior and inferior to the mastoid process.
4. Yifeng (TE 17): Posterior to the lobule of the ear, in the depression between the mandible and mastoid process.
5. Qimai (TE 18): In the center of the mastoid process, at the junction of the middle and lower third of the curve formed by Yifeng (TE 17) and Jiaosun (TE 20) posterior to the helix.
6. Luxi (TE 19): Posterior to the ear, at the junction of the upper and middle third of the curve formed by Yifeng (TE 17) and Jiaosun (TE 20) behind the helix.
7. Jiaosun (TE 20): Directly above the ear apex, within the hair-line.
8. Erheliao (TE 22): Anterior and superior to Ermen (TE 21), at the level with the root of the auricle, on the posterior border of the hairline of the temple where the superficial temporal artery passes.

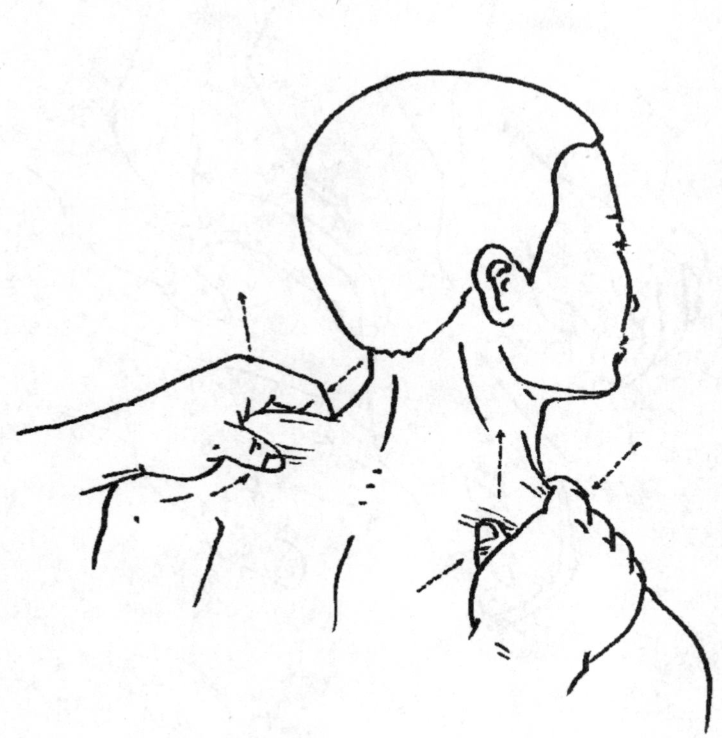

Holding technique on Jianjing (GB 21).

Manipulation

Place two thumbs respectively below Jianjing (GB 21) and other fingers at the front of the shoulder. Then grasp and lift the shoulder muscles with wrist strength 3-5 times, each time should last 10-20 seconds.

Points

Jianjing (GB 21): Midway between the lower border of the spinous process of the seventh cervical vertebra and the acromion.

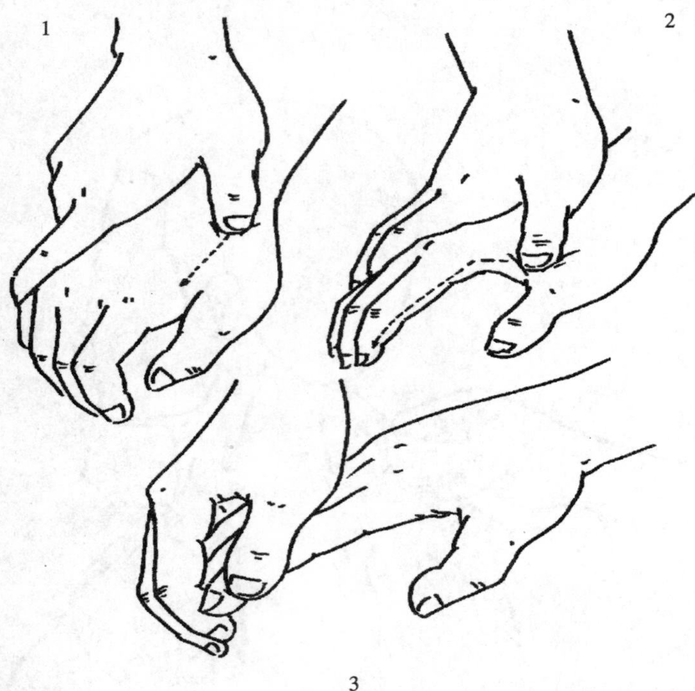

Kneading technique on Hegu (LI 4).

Manipulation

Place a thumb on Yangxi (LI 5) located at the wrist and lay other four fingers at the side of the hand. Then push downwards from Yangxi (LI 5) along the side of the index finger to Hegu (LI 4) as shown in figure 2, knead Hegu (LI 4) for 10-30 seconds and push to Shangyang (LI 1). Repeat the manipulation for 3-5 times.

Points

1. Yangxi (LI 5): On the radial side of the wrist, in the depression between the tendons of m. extensor pollicis longus and brevis.

2. Hegu (LI 4): On the dorsum of the hand, between the first and second metacarpal bones, approximately in the middle of the second metacarpal bone on the radial side.

3. Shangyang (LI 1): On the radial side of the index finger, about 0.1 *cun* posterior to the corner of the nail.

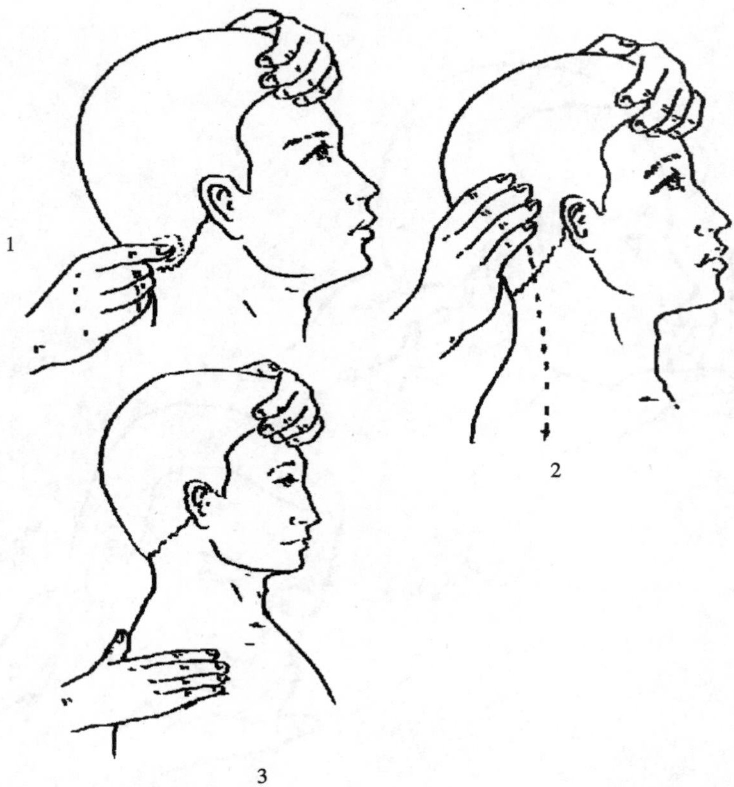

Stationary circular pressing technique on Fengchi (GB 20).

Manipulation

1. Place one hand on the front of forehead to keep it still and then knead Fengchi (GB 20) with the thumb and index finger of the other hand for 1-3 minutes.

2. Place four finger-pulps of one hand at Naokong (GB 19), then push and rub downwards past Fengchi (GB 20) and stop at Jianjing (GB 21), (See figures 2 and 3). Repeat the massage at each side for 1-3 minutes.

Points

1. Fengchi (GB 20): In the depression between the upper portion of m. sternocleidomastoideus and m. trapezius, on the same level with Fengfu (GV16).

2. Naokong (GB 19): 1.5 *cun* above Fengchi (GB 20).

3. Jianjing (GB 21): Midway between the lower border of the spinous process of the seventh cervical vertebra and the acromion.

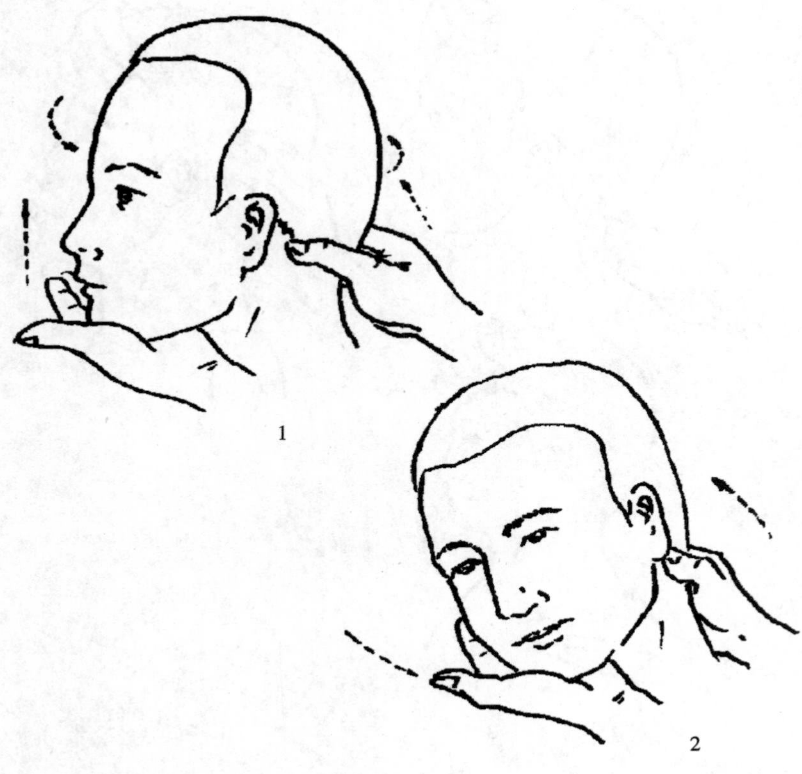

1

2

Neck rotation technique.

Manipulation

Hold the mandibule with one palm and place the other hand on the nape, then gently knead the neck muscles for 1-3 minutes. Then pull up the chin slightly and rotate the neck leftward and rightward gently a few times; then suddenly turn the head leftward or rightward, meanwhile a click may be heard, which should not be enforced. By now the manipulation is over.

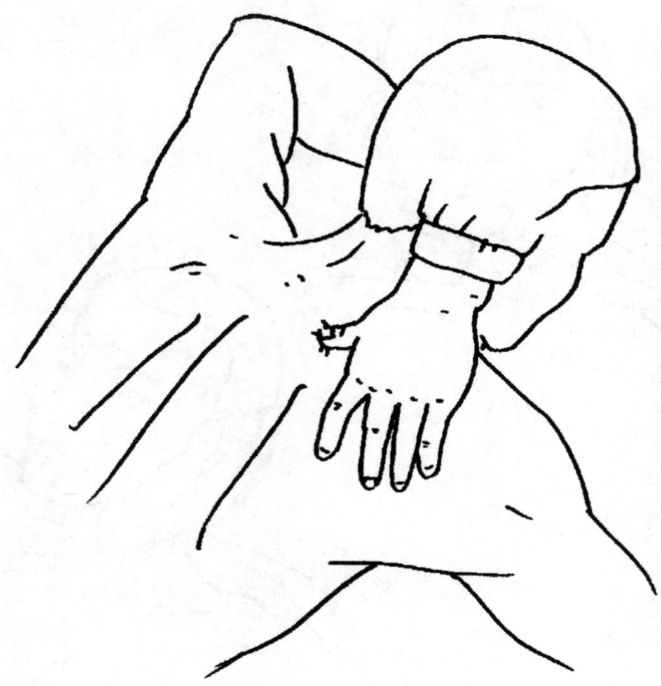

Finger stationary circular pressing technique on Quyuan (SI 13).

Manipulation

Place one thumb on Quyuan (SI 13) of the affected side while other four fingers on the back of the shoulder as shown in the picture. Knead Quyuan (SI 13) with the thumb for 3-5 minutes.

Points

Quyuan (SI 13): On the medial extremity of the suprascapular fossa, at the level of the spinous process of the second thoracic vertebra.

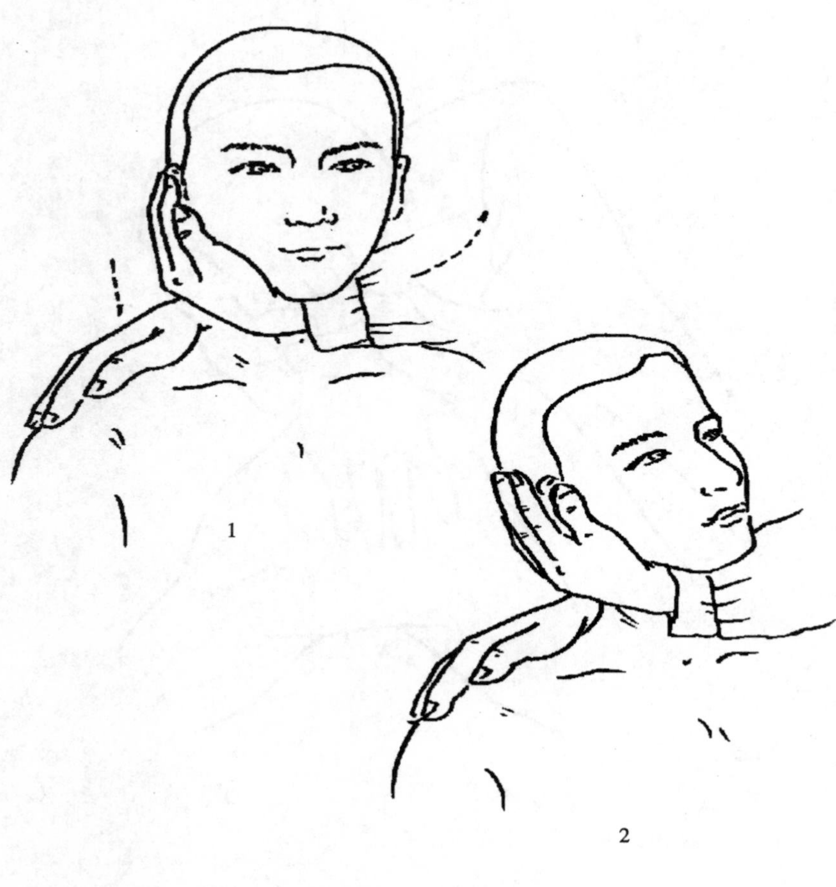

Neck rotation while pressing the shoulder technique.

Manipulation

Place one palm, by passing the nape, on the shoulder. Let the other hand go through the front of head to hold it steadily, then turn the neck towards one side and slightly pull it in an outward and upward direction. Repeat the manipulation for 1-2 minutes.

Scapulohumeral Periarthritis

Clinical Manifestations

The disease is marked by soreness, distention and pain of the soft tissue in one or both shoulders with limitation of movement. The pain is increased and radiates towards the neck and upper limbs, when the patient makes internal or external rotation or abduction to a certain degree. The pain is static in nature, mild during the day and severe at night. The patient is often woken up at night by the severe pain, which may be alleviated by gentle exercise in the morning.

Differentiation of syndromes:

A. Cold Bi syndrome: Severe cold pain at the shoulder, aggravated by exposure to wind or cold and alleviated by warmth; the pain is fixed in location without local redness, heat, or swelling. Pale tongue with thin and white coating, wiry and tense pulse.

B. Damp Bi syndrome: Soreness, heaviness and pain of the shoulder with muscle numbness; heavy and weak extremities with limited movement of the joint. Pale tongue with white coating, soft and slow pulse.

Treatment Principle

Removing the obstruction from the meridian and collateral and smoothing the joint.

Tuina Techniques

A. Rubbing and pressing techniques around the shoulder.

B. Holding technique on Jianjing (GB 21).

C. Pushing and pressing techniques on the three points of Yangming meridian.

D. Shoulder traction technique.

E. Pressing technique on Jiquan (HT 1).

Addition or Subtraction Techniques

A. Cold Bi syndrome:

Addition: 1. Pressing technique around the shoulder. 2. Shoulder rotation technique.

B. Damp Bi syndrome:

Addition: 1. Holding and lifting techniques around the shoulder. 2. Pressing technique on Quepen (ST 12).

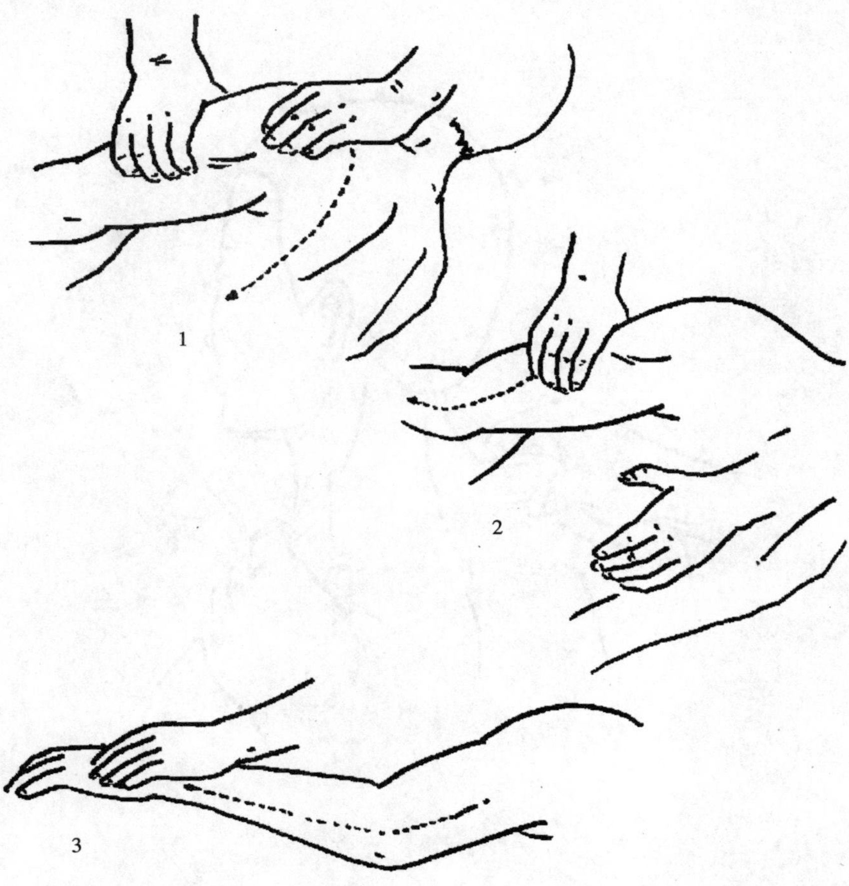

Rubbing and pressing techniques around the shoulder.

Manipulation

Place two palms on the lower end of the neck, rub and press respectively along the acromion and the scapular region for 2-5 minutes. Then from the acromion massage down to the elbow and the wrist for 2-5 minutes.

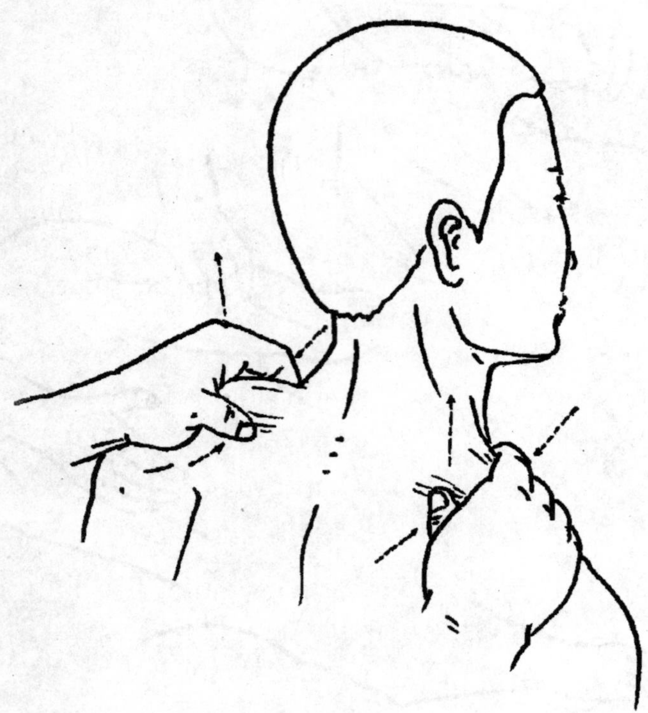

Holding technique on Jianjing (GB 21).

Manipulation

Place two thumbs respectively below Jianjing (GB 21). Place other fingers at the front of the shoulder. Then grasp and lift the shoulder muscles with wrist strength 3-5 times, each time should last 10-20 seconds.

Points

Jianjing (GB 21): Midway between the lower border of the spinous process of the seventh cervical vertebra and the acromion.

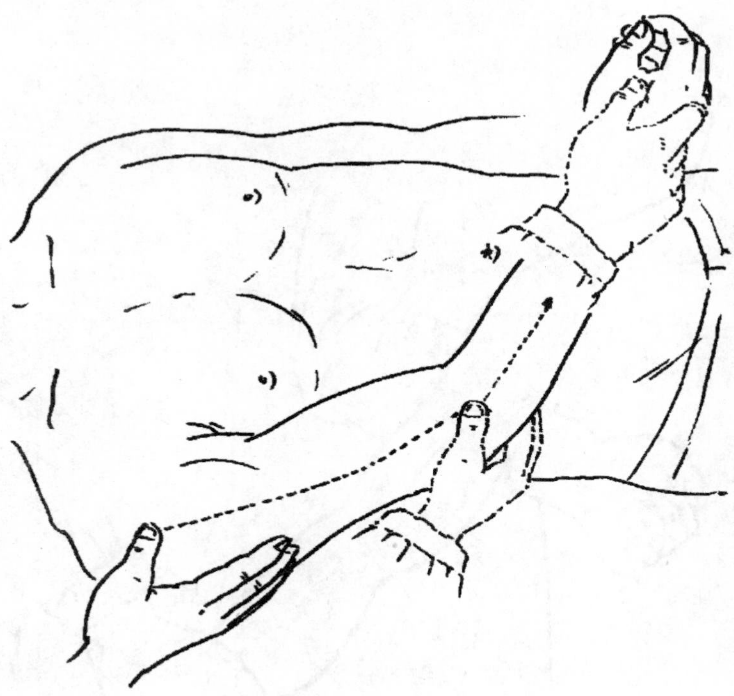

Pushing and pressing techniques on the three points of Yangming Meridian.

Manipulation

Place a thumb on Jianyu (LI 15), then push downwards along the affected arm, pass Quchi (LI 11) and stop at Hegu (LI 4). Repeat the manipulation for 1-3 minutes.

Points

1. Jianyu (LI 15): In the depression appearing at the anterior border of the acromioclavicular joint when the arm is in full abduction.

2. Quchi (LI 11): In the depression at the lateral end of the transverse cubital crease.

3. Hegu (LI 4): On the dorsum of the hand, between the first and second metacarpal bones, approximately in the middle of the second metacarpal bone on the radial side.

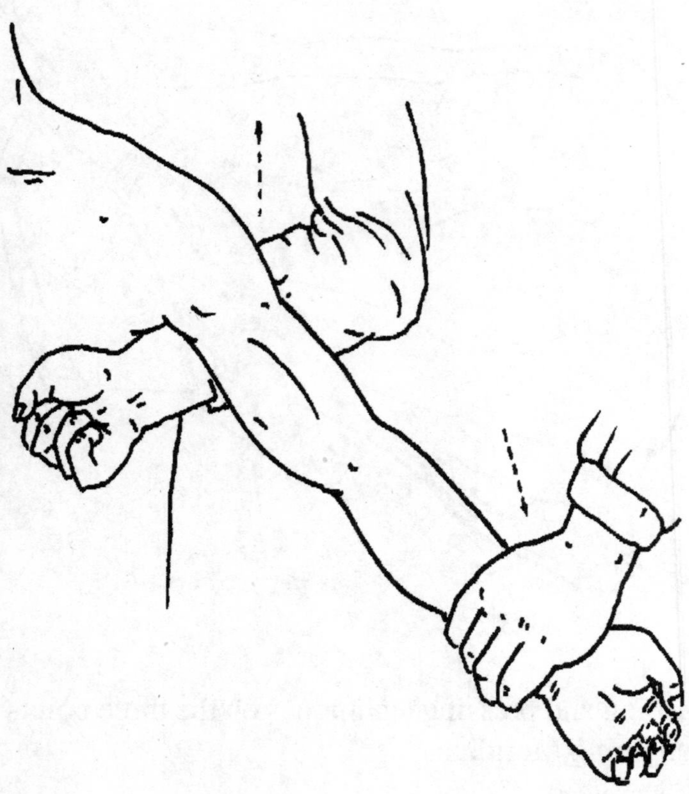

Shoulder traction technique.

Manipulation

Insert one forearm underneath the armpit, let the other hand grab the wrist. Use forearm to lift up the arm while using the other hand to push down and stretch the shoulder region at a slightly diagonal angle. Repeat the manipulation for 3-5 times, each time 30-60 seconds.

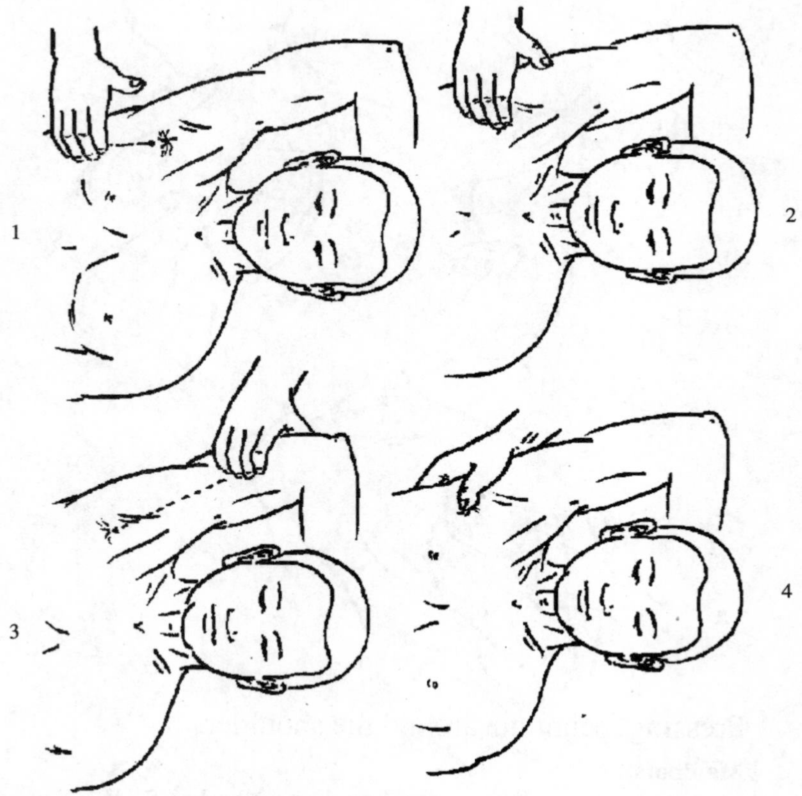

Pressing technique on Jiquan (HT 1).

Manipulation

Place four fingers on Yuanye (GB 22), and rub upwards to Jiquan (HT 1), then place the four fingers on Qingling (HT 2) and rub downwards to Jiquan (HT 1). Repeat each manipulation for 1-2 minutes. Then place the thumbs on Jiquan (HT 1) while other fingers wrap around the back of the shoulder, and then press Jiquan (HT 1) for 2-3 times, each time should last 30-60 seconds.

Points

1. Yuanye (GB 22): On the mid-axillary line, in the fourth intercostal space.
2. Qingling (HT 2): 3 *cun* directly above the medial end of the transverse cubital crease.
3. Jiquan (HT 1): In the center of the axilla, on the medial side of the axillary artery.

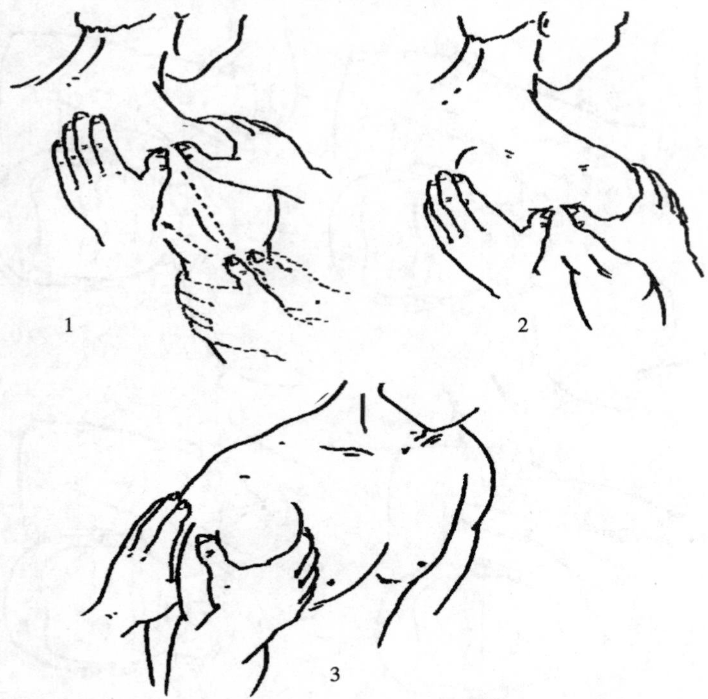

Pressing technique around the shoulder.

Manipulation

Place two thumbs at a diagonal angle on Naoshu (SI 10), then move diagonally down to Binao (LI 14), and Jianzhen (SI 9). Lastly, place one thumb on Jiquan (HT 1), while other four fingers on Zhongfu (LU 1) and Yunmen (LU 2). Press and knead each point for 30-60 seconds. Repeat the manipulation 2-3 times.

Points

1. Naoshu (SI 10): Directly above the posterior end of the axillary fold, in the depression inferior to the scapular spine.

2. Binao (LI 14): 7 *cun* directly above the lateral end of the transverse cubital crease, superior to the lower end of m. deltoideus.

3. Jianzhen (SI 9): 1 *cun* directly above the posterior end of the axillary fold.

4. Jiquan (HT 1): In the center of the axilla, on the medial side of the axillary artery.

5. Zhongfu (LU1): 6 *cun* lateral to the anterior midline, at the level of the first intercostal space.

6. Yunmen (LU2): 6 *cun* lateral to the anterior midline, at the lower border of the clavicle.

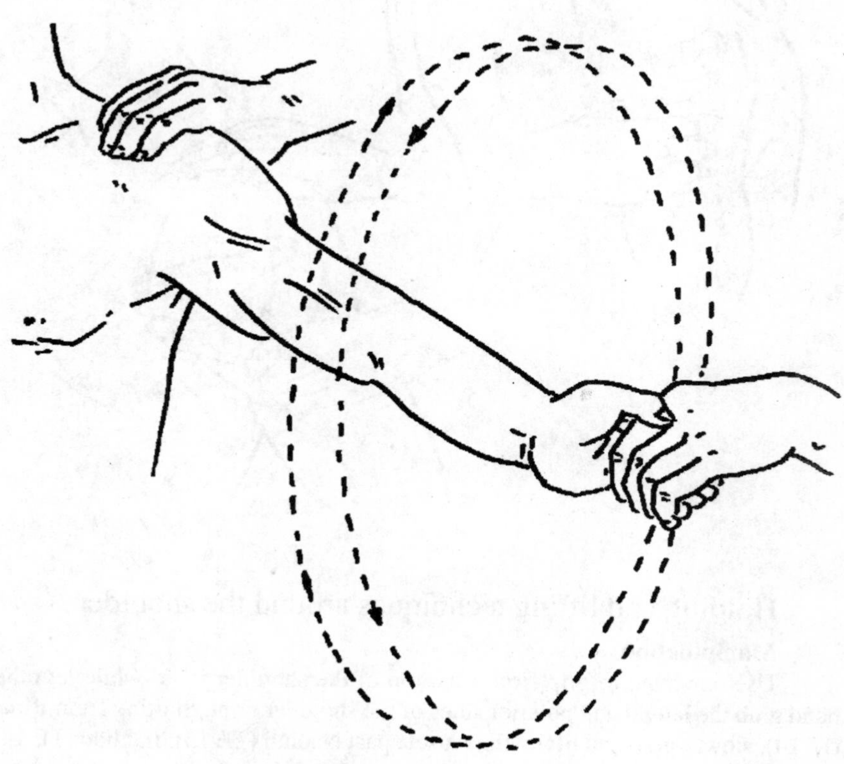

Shoulder rotation technique.

Manipulation

Place one hand on the shoulder and let the other hand grab the patient's fingers and then rotate the arm clockwise and counterclockwise. Repeat circular movement of the arm in each direction 10-20 times.

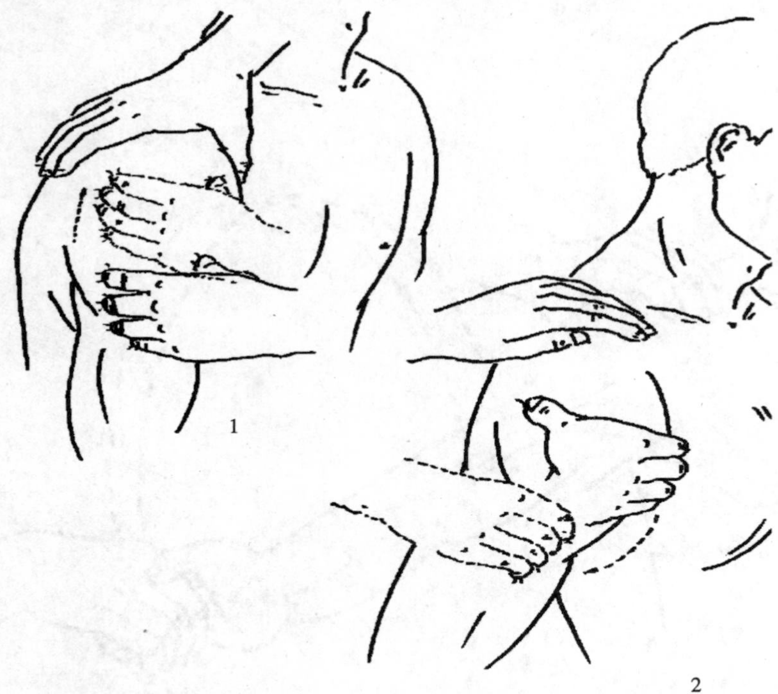

Holding and lifting techniques around the shoulder.

Manipulation

Use one hand to grip firmly the top of the shoulder joint, while let other hand grab the lateral and poterior sides of the shoulder joint. Starting from Binao (LI 14), slowly grab and lift up the muscle past Naohui (TE 13), Jianliao (TE 14), and stop at Jianyu (LI 15), repeat 1-2 minutes. Then place the hand on the anterior inferior border of the deltoid muscle, grab and lift the muscle to Binao (LI 14), repeat the manipulation for 2-3 minutes.

Points

1. Binao (LI 14): 7 *cun* directly above the lateral end of the transverse cubital crease, superior to the lower end of m. deltoideus.

2. Naohui (TE 13): In the depression about 3 *cun* directly down to the posterior and inferior of the acromion, on the posterior border of m. deltoideus.

3. Jianliao (TE 14): In the posterior depression of the acromion when the arm is abducted.

4. Jianyu (LI 15): In the anterior depression of the acromion when the arm is abducted.

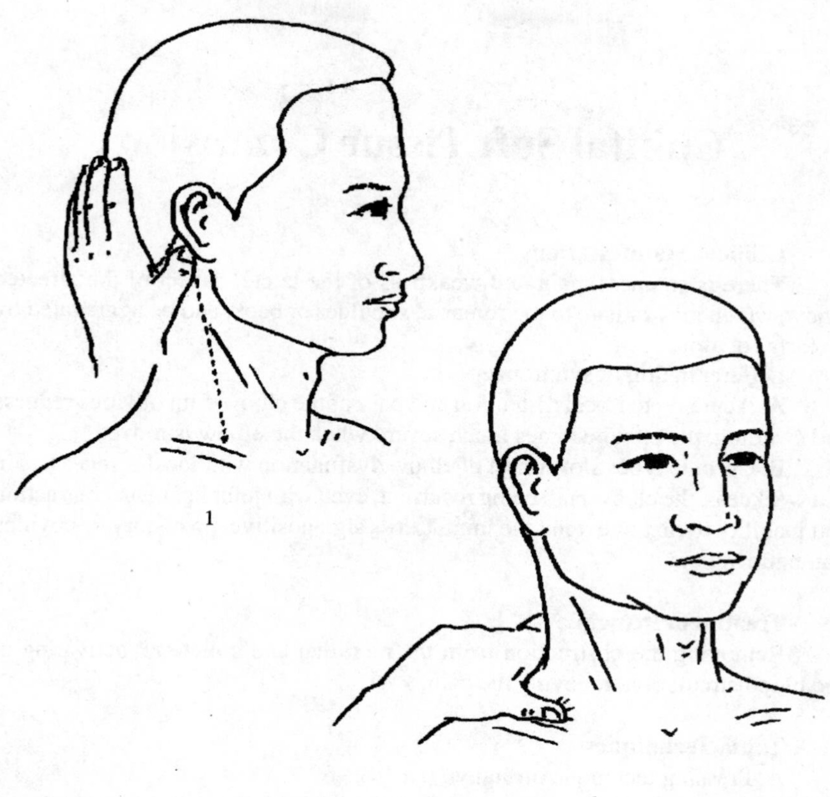

Pressing technique on Quepen (ST 12).

Manipulation

Place a thumb on Yifeng (TE 17), and then rub along the sternocleidomastoid muscle to Quepen (ST 12). Perform the manipulation 5-10 times. Then press Quepen (ST 12) 2-3 times, each time should last 15-30 seconds.

Points

1. Yifeng (TE 17): Posterior to the lobule of the ear, in the depression between the mandible and mastoid process.
2. Quepen (ST 12): In the midpoint of the supraclavicular fossa, 4 *cun* lateral to the anterior midline.

Cubital Soft Tissue Contusion

Clinical Manifestations

There is soreness, pain and weakness of the lateral aspect of the affected elbow, which may radiate to the forearm, shoulder or back, and be aggravated by forearm rotation.

Differentiation of syndromes:

A. Acute type: Local distention and pain of the elbow with obvious redness and swelling, the pain becomes much severe when the elbow is moved.

B. Chronic type: Slow onset of elbow dysfunction with local soreness, pain and weakness, the elbow pain being recurrent, even with joint ligament contraction and inability to flex or extend the joint. Leri's sign positive, no history of obvious traumatic injury.

Treatment Principle

Removing the obstruction from the meridian and collateral, activating qi and blood circulation, relieving the pain.

Tuina Techniques

A. Pressing technique on Jianyu (LI 14).

B. Pushing technique along the three Yang meridians of Hand on the upper arm.

C. Pushing technique along the three Yin meridians of Hand on the upper arm.

D. Pushing technique along the three Yin meridians of Hand on the forearm.

E. Pressing technique on Jiquan (HT 1).

Addition or Subtraction Techniques

A. Acute type: Tuina treatment can be given only 2-3 days after the contusion.

Addition: 1. Pinching technique along the upper arm. 2. Pushing technique along the three Yang meridians of Hand on the forearm.

B. Chronic type:

Addition: 1. Pressing technique on Jugu (LI 16). 2. Combing technique on the dorsum of the hand.

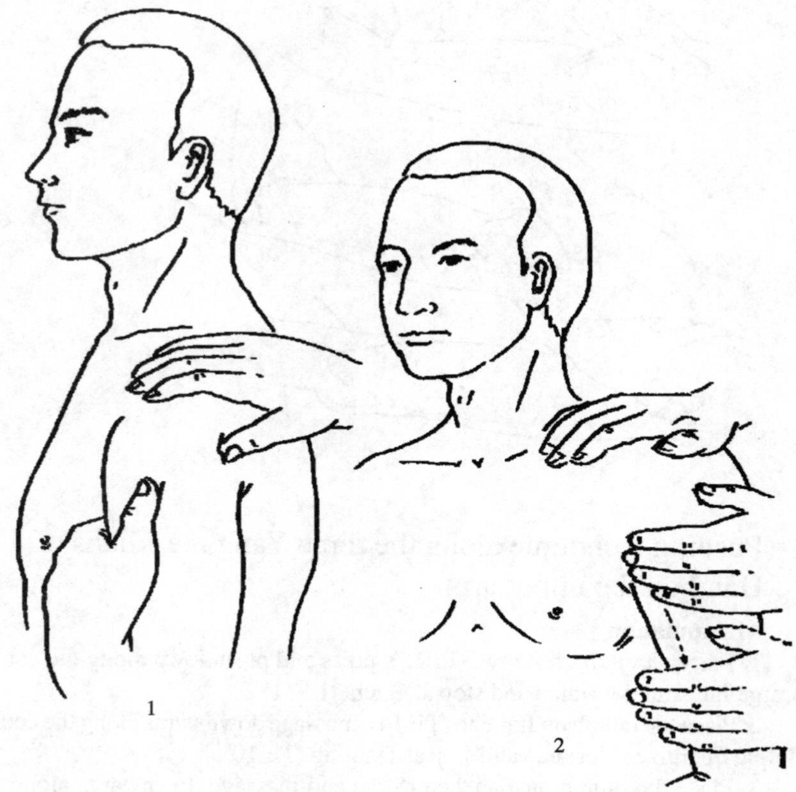

Pressing technique on Jianyu (LI 15).

Manipulation

Place a thumb on Jianyu (LI 15) and let other four fingers hold the shoulder joint. Press and knead Jianyu (LI 15) with the thumb for 1-2 minutes. Withdraw the thumb , then place the other palm on Jianyu (LI 15), push and rub down to Binao (LI 14). Repeat the massage for 1-2 minutes.

Points

1. Jianyu (LI 15): In the anterior depression of the acromion when the arm is abducted.

2. Binao (LI 14): 7 *cun* directly above the lateral end of the transverse cubital crease, superior to the lower end of m. deltoideus.

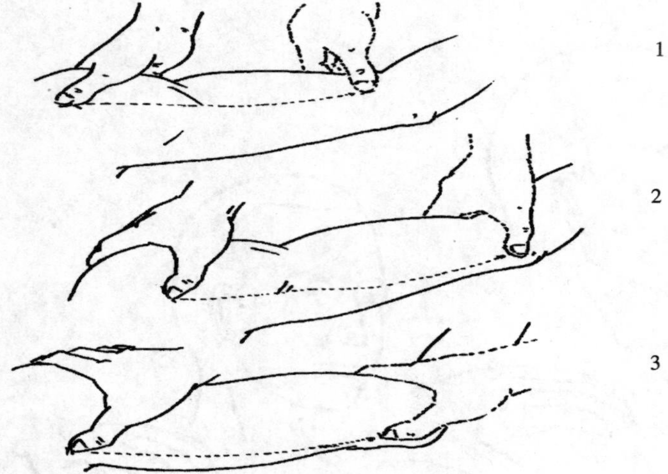

Pushing technique along the three Yang meridians of Hand on the upper arm.

Manipulation

1. Place a thumb on Jianyu (LI 15), press and push down along the course of Large Intestine Meridian and stop at Quchi (LI 11).

2. Place the thumb on Jianliao (TE 14), massage downwards along the course of Triple Energizer Meridian and stop at Tianjing (TE 10).

3. Place the thumb on Jianzhen (SI 9) and massage downwards along the course of Small Intestine Meridian down to Xiaohai (SI 8).

Repeat the manipulation on each meridian for 1-2 minutes.

Points

1. Jianyu (LI 15): In the anterior depression of the acromion when the arm is abducted.

2. Quchi (LI 11): In the depression at the lateral end of the transverse cubital crease. (He-Sea Point).

3. Jianliao (TE 14): In the posterior depression of the acromion when the arm is abducted.

4. Tianjing (TE 10): In the depression about 1 *cun* superior to the olecranon. (He-Sea Point).

5. Jianzhen (SI 9): 1 *cun* above the posterior end of the axillary fold.

6. Xiaohai (SI 8): In the depression between the olecranon of the ulna and the medial epicondyle of the humerus. (He-Sea Point).

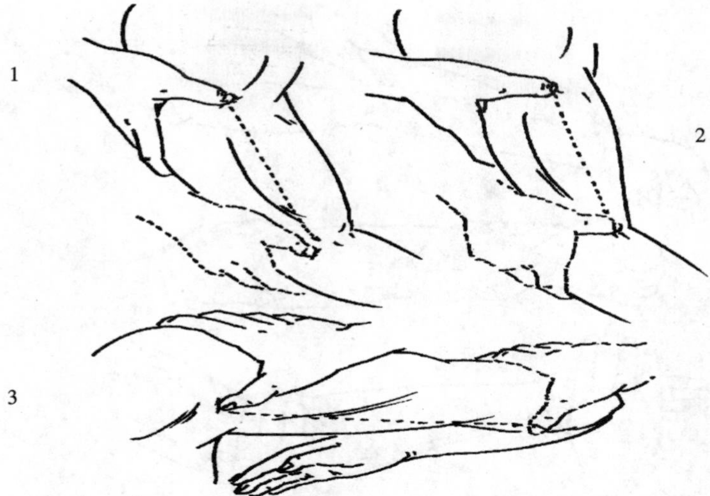

Pushing technique along the three Yin meridians of Hand on the upper arm.

Manipulation

1. Place a thumb on Tianfu (LU 3), press and push down along the Lung Meridian and stop at Chize (LU 5).

2. Place the thumb on Tianquan (PC 2), massage downwards along the Pericardium Meridian and stop at Quze (PC 3).

3. Place the thumb on Jiquan (HT 1) and massage downwards along the Heart Meridian down to Shaohai (HT 3).

Repeat the manipulation on each meridian for 1-2 minutes.

Points

1. Tianfu (LU 3): On the medial aspect of the upper arm, 3 *cun* below the end of the axillary fold, on the radial side of m. biceps brachii.

2. Chize (LU 5): On the cubital crease, on the radial side of the tendon of m. biceps brachii. (He-Sea Point).

3. Tianquan (PC 2): 2 *cun* below the level of the anterior axillary fold, between the two heads of m. biceps brachii.

4. Quze (PC 3): On the transverse cubital crease, at the ulnar side of the tendon of m. biceps brachii. (He-Sea Point).

5. Jiquan (HT 1): In the center of the axilla, on the medial side of the axillary artery.

6. Shaohai (HT 3): When the elbow is flexed, the point is at the mid-point of the line jointing the medial end of the transverse cubital crease and the medial epicondyle of the humerus.

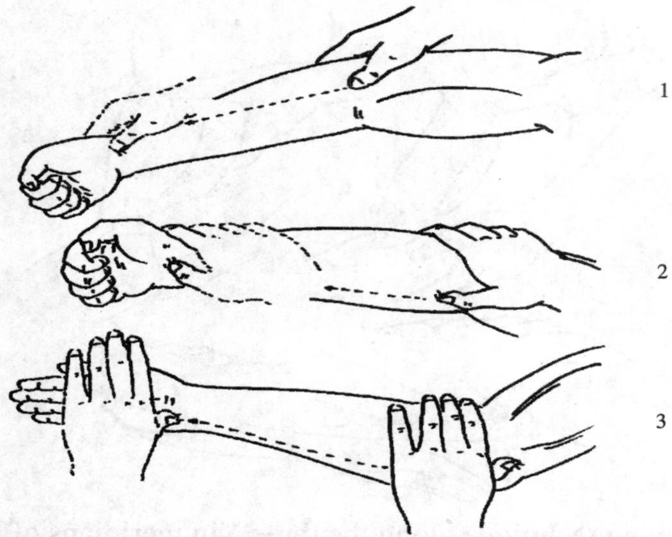

Pushing technique along the three Yin meridians of Hand on forearm.

Manipulation

Place one thumb on Chize (LU 5), press and push down to Taiyuan (LU 9) along the course of the lung meridian. Then place the thumb on Quze (PC 3) and press and push along the course of the pericardium meridian down to Daling (PC 7), then lay the thumb on Shaohai (HT 3), push and press down to Shenmen (HT 7) following the heart meridian. Repeat the manipulation on each meridian for 1-2 minutes.

Points

1. Chize (LU 5): On the cubital crease, on the radial side of the tendon of m. biceps brachii. (He-sea point).

2. Taiyuan (LU 9): At the radial end of the transverse crease of the wrist, in the depression on the lateral side of the radial artery. (Shu-stream point).

3. Quze (PC 3): On the transverse cubital crease, at the ulnar side of the tendon of m. biceps brachii. (He-sea point).

4. Daling (PC 7): In the middle of the transverse crease of the wrist, between the tendons of m. palmaris longus and m. flexor carpi radialis. (Shu-stream point).

5. Shaohai (HT 3): When the elbow is flexed into a right angle, the point is in the depression between the medial end of the transverse cubital crease and the medial epicondyle of the humerus.

6. Shenmen (HT 7): At the ulnar end of the transverse crease of the wrist, in the depression on the radial side of the tendon of m. flexor carpi ulnaris.

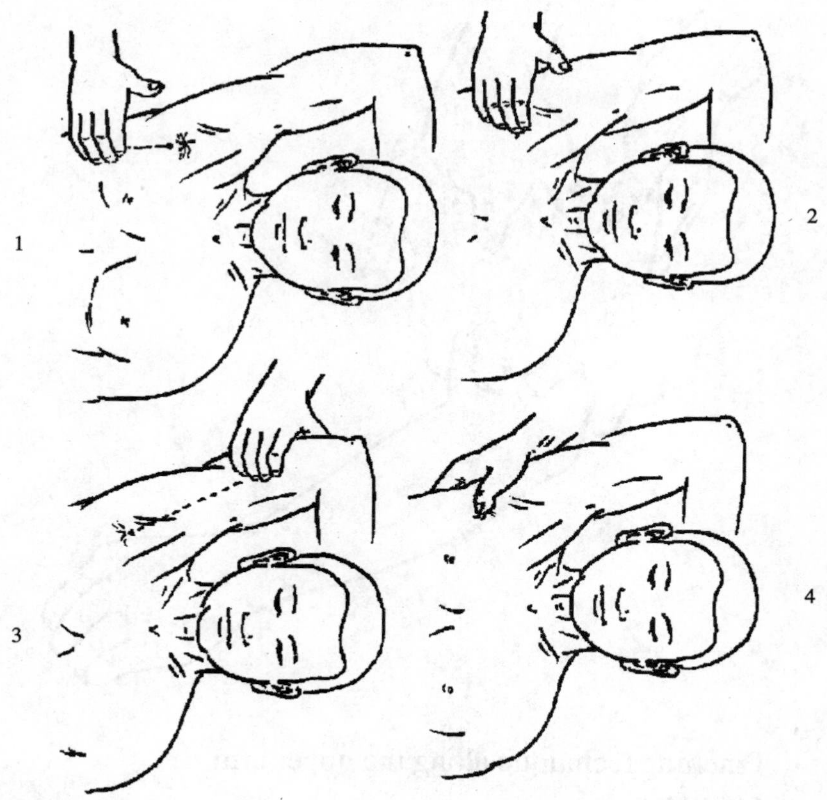

Pressing technique on Jiquan (HT 1).

Manipulation

Place four fingers on Yuanye (GB 22), and rub upwards to Jiquan (HT 1), then place the fingers on Qingling (HT 2) and rub to Jiquan (HT 1). Repeat each manipulation for 1-2 minutes. Then place the thumbs on Jiquan (HT 1) and let other fingers wrap around the back of the shoulder. Press Jiquan (HT 1) 2-3 times, each time should last 30-60 seconds.

Points

1. Yuanye (GB 22): On the mid-axillary line, in the fourth intercostal space.
2. Qingling (HT 2): 3 *cun* directly above the medial end of the transverse cubital crease.
3. Jiquan (HT 1): In the center of the axilla, on the medial side of the axillary artery.

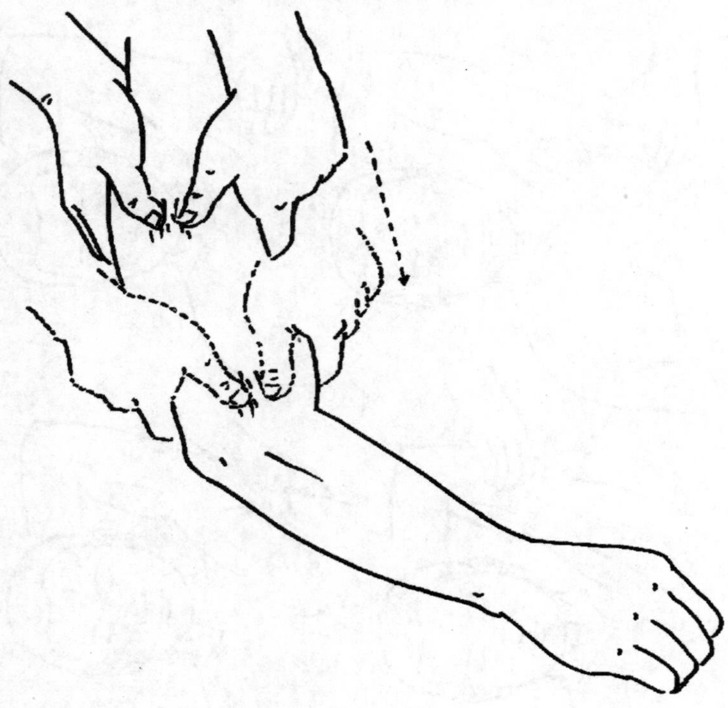

Pinching technique along the upper arm.

Manipulation

Place two thumb tips on Binao (LI 14) and let other finger-pulps touch Jiquan (HT 1) on the armpit. Pinch and press Binao (LI 14) for 1-2 minutes. Then massage from Binao (LI 14) downwards to Quchi (LI 11) and Shaohai (HT 3) by pushing technique, press and knead these two acupoints for 30-60 seconds. Repeat the manipulation for 3-5 times.

Points

1. Binao (LI 14): 7 *cun* directly above the lateral end of the transverse cubital crease, superior to the lower end of m. deltoideus.

2. Jiquan (HT 1): In the center of the axilla, on the medial side of the axillary artery.

3. Quchi (LI 11): In the depression at the lateral end of the transverse cubital crease. (He-Sea Point).

4. Shaohai (HT 3): When the elbow is flexed, the point is at the mid-point of the line jointing the medial end of the transverse cubital crease and the medial epicondyle of the humerus.

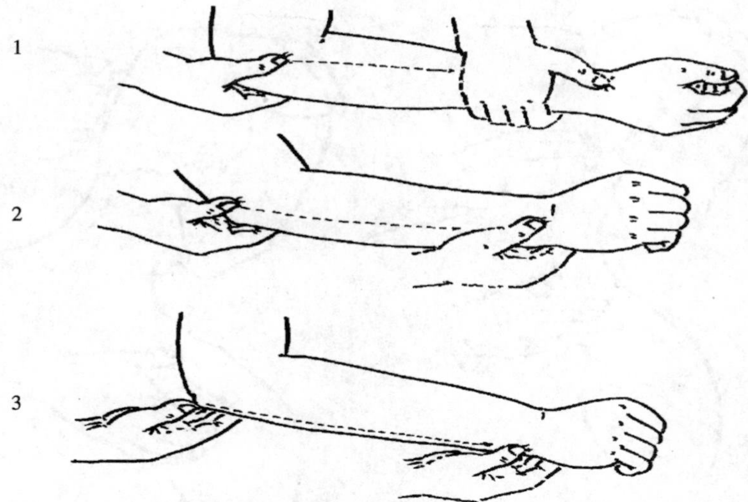

Pushing technique along the three Yang meridians of Hand on the forearm.

Manipulation

Place a thumb on Quchi (LI 11), Tianjing (TE 10),and Xiaohai (SI 8) respectively, push and press downwards (along the Large Intestine Meridian, Triple Energizer Meridian, and the Small Intestine Meridian respectively) to Yangxi (LI 5), Yangchi (TE 4), and Yanggu (SI 5). Repeat the manipulation on each meridian for 1-2 minutes.

Points

1. Quchi (LI 11): In the depression at the lateral end of the transverse cubital crease. (He-Sea Point).

2. Yangxi (LI 5): On the radial side of the transverse crease of the wrist, in the depression between the tendons of m. extensor pollicis longus and brevis. (Jing-River Point).

3. Tianjing (TE 10): In the depression about 1 *cun* superior to the olecranon. (He-Sea Point).

4. Yangchi (TE 4): On the transverse crease of the dorsum of wrist, in the depression lateral to the tendon of m. extensor digitorum communis. (Yuan-Primary Point).

5. Xiaohai (SI 8): In the depression between the olecranon of the ulna and the medial epicondyle of the humerus. (He-Sea Point).

6. Yanggu (SI 5): At the ulnar end of the transverse crease on the dorsal aspect of the wrist, in the depression between the styloid process of the ulna and the triquetral bone (Jing-River Point).

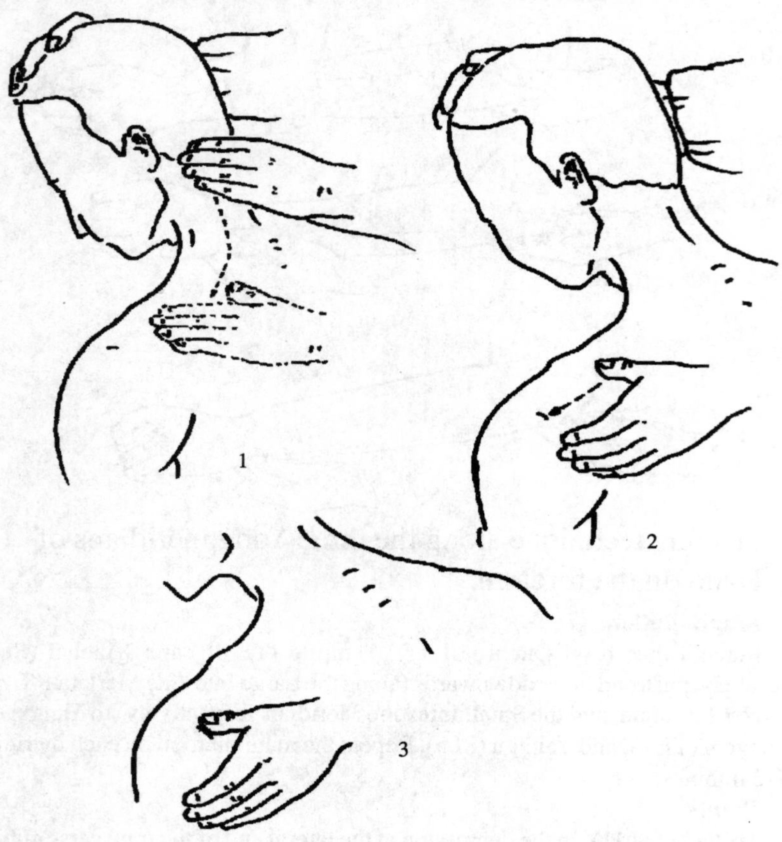

Pressing technique on Jugu (LI 16).

Manipulation

Place four finger-pulps just under the posterior hairline of the affected side of the head and rub down along the neck and shoulder past Wangu (GB 12), Jianjing (GB 21) to Jugu (LI 16). Repeat rubbing for 1-2 minutes. Then place the thumb on Jianjing (GB 21), and rub to Jugu (LI 16), then knead for 1-2 minutes.

Points

1. Wangu (GB 12): In the depression posterior and inferior to the mastoid process.

2. Jianjing (GB 21): Midway between the seventh cervical vertebra and the acromion.

3. Jugu (LI 16): In the depression between the acromial extremity of the clavicle and the scapular spine.

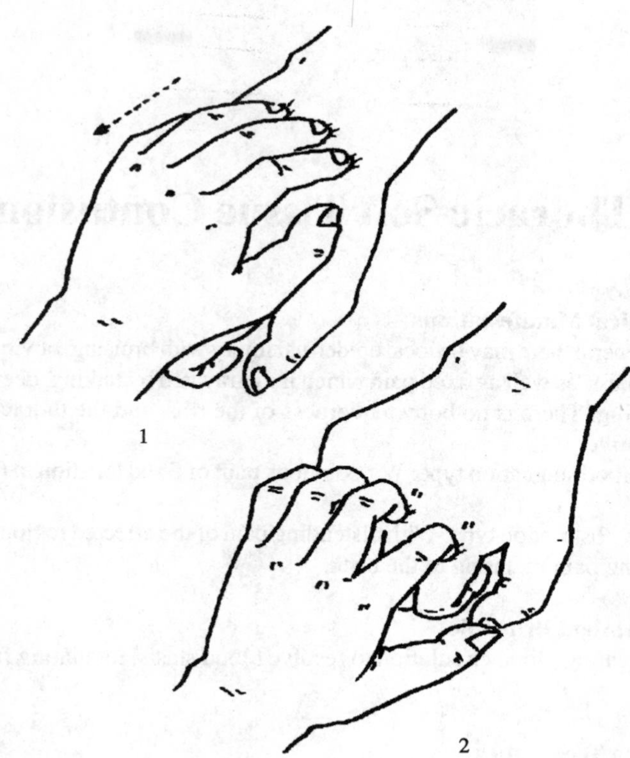

Combing technique on the dorsum of the hand.

Manipulation

Place four finger-pulps at the level of Yangchi (TE 4), then comb downwards along the interspaces between metacarple bones and stop at Yemen (TE 2). Repeat the manipulation for 3-5 minutes.

Points

1. Yangchi (TE 4): On the transverse crease of the dorsum of wrist, in the depression lateral to the tendon of m. extensor digitorum communis.

2. Yemen (TE 2): In the depression proximal to the margin of the web between the ring finger and small finger.

Thoracic Soft Tissue Contusion

Clinical Manifestations

In general there may be local epidermal injury with bruising, obvious swelling and tenderness, as well as fixed pain which is aggravated by talking, deep breathing and coughing. There is no bony tenderness of the ribs, and the thoracic pressing test is negative.

A. Blood stagnation type: With obvious pain of fixed location in the affected region.

B. *Qi* obstruction type: With distending pain of the affected region, combined with burning pain radiating to the back.

Treatment Principle

Activating blood circulation to resolve blood stasis, regulating flow of *qi* to stop pain.

Tuina Techniques

A. Rubbing chest technique.

B. Rubbing the intercostal spaces technique.

C. Pressing technique on Zhongfu (LU 1) and Yunmen (LU 2).

D. Digital pressing technique on the chest and abdomen.

E. Finger stationary circular pressing technique on Quyuan (SI 13).

F. Chest stretching technique.

G. Opposite pressing technique on Neiguan (PC 6) and Waiguan (TE 5).

Addition or Subtraction Techniques

A. Blood stagnation type:

Addition: 1. Pinching technique on the anterior of the axilla. 2. Pressing technique on Quepen (ST 12).

B. *Qi* obstruction type:

Addition: 1. Digital pressing technique on the back. 2. Holding and lifting techniques on the back.

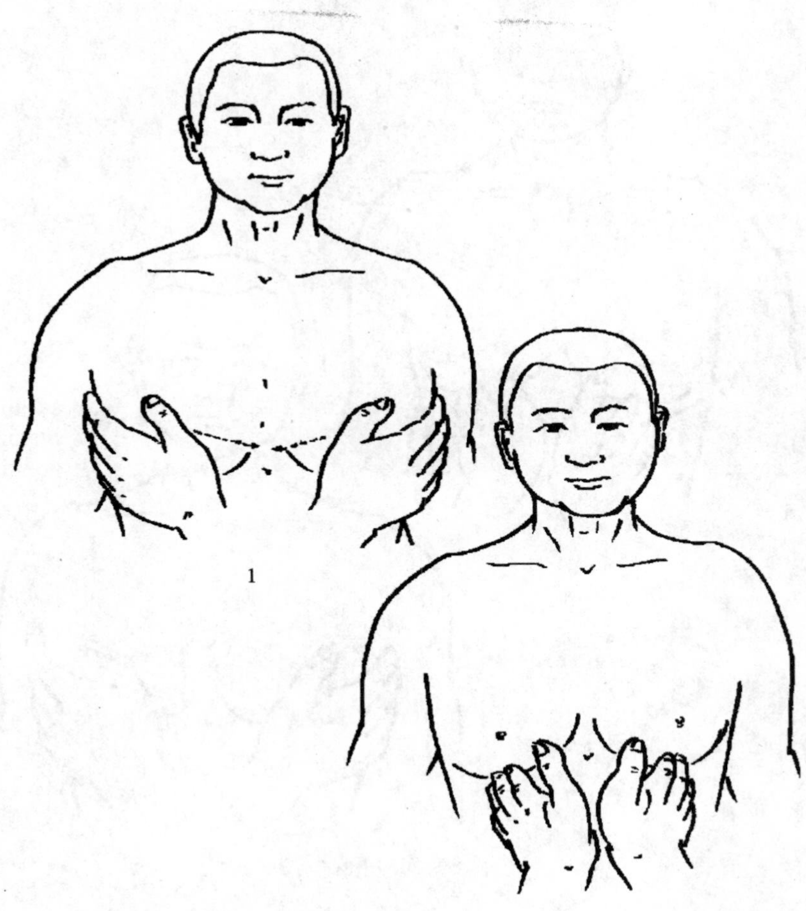

1

2

Rubbing chest technique.

Manipulation

Place two palms respectively on bilateral Yuanye (GB 22) and Dabao (SP 21) with fingers touching the intercostal spaces. Massage from Yuanye (GB 22) and Dabao (SP 21) to Qimen (LR 14) as shown in figure 1 and 2. Repeat the manipulation for 1-3 minutes.

Points

1. Yuanye (GB 22): On the mid-axillary line, in the fourth intercostal space.
2. Dabao (SP 21): On the mid-axillary line, in the sixth intercostal space.
3. Qimen (LR 14): Directly below the nipple, in the sixth intercostal space.

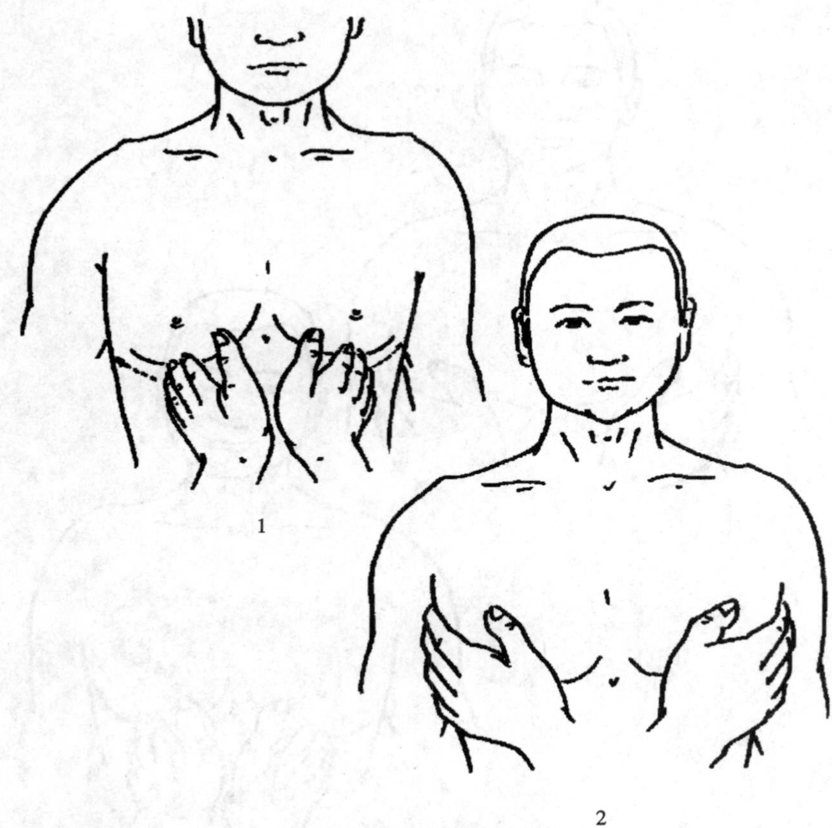

1

2

Rubbing the intercostal spaces technique.

Manipulation

Place four fingertips of both hands respectively on Qimen (LR 14) and Riyue (GB 24), massage laterally along the intercostal spaces to the two sides of the chest, to Yuanye (GB 22) and Dabao (SP 21). Repeat the manipulation for 1-3 minutes.

Points

1. Qimen (LR 14): Directly below the nipple, in the sixth intercostal space.
2. Riyue (GB 24): Directly below the nipple, in the seventh intercostal space.
3. Yuanye (GB 22): On the mid-axillary line, in the fourth intercostal space.
4. Dabao (SP 21): On the mid-axillary line, in the sixth intercostal space.

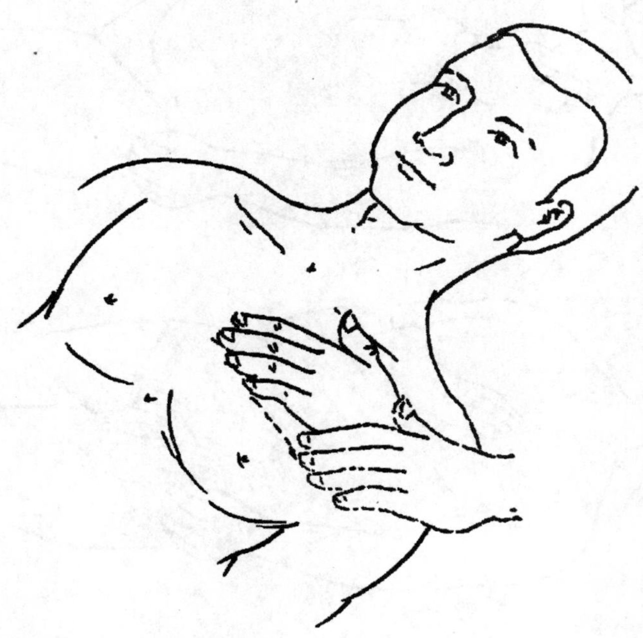

Pressing technique on Zhongfu (LU 1) and Yunmen (LU 2).

Manipulation

With fingers slightly apart from one another, place four fingertips of one hand on the medial border of musculus pectoralis major, then rub horizontally along the intercostal spaces across the chest to Zhongfu (LU 1) and Yunmen (LU 2). Repeat the massage 2-5 times, each time should last 15-30 seconds.

Points

1. Zhongfu (LU 1): 6 *cun* lateral to the anterior midline, at the level of the first intercostal space.

2. Yunmen (LU 2): In the depression below the acromial extremity of the clavicle, 6 *cun* lateral to the anterior midline.

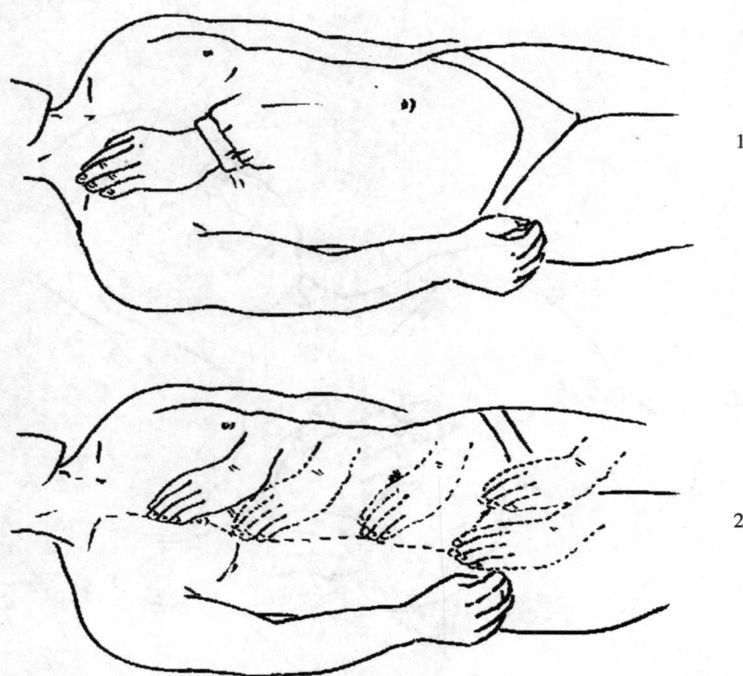

Digital pressing technique on chest and abdomen.

Manipulation

Place four fingertips of one hand on Qihu (ST 13), then slowly press the intercostal space downwards along Yingchuang (ST 16), Qimen (LR 14), Daheng (SP 15), Fushe (SP 13), and stop at Qichong (ST 30). Repeat the manipulation 2-3 times.

Points

1. Qihu (ST 13): At the lower border of the clavicle, 4 *cun* lateral to the anterior midline.
2. Yingchuang (ST 16): In the third intercostal space, 4 *cun* lateral to the anterior midline.
3. Qimen (LR 14): Directly below the nipple, in the sixth intercostal space.
4. Daheng (SP 15): 4 *cun* lateral to the center of the umbilicus.
5. Fushe (SP 13): 3.5 *cun* below the center of the umbilicus and 4 *cun* lateral to the anterior midline.
6. Qichong (ST 30): 5 *cun* below the center of the umbilicus and 2 *cun* lateral to the anterior midline.

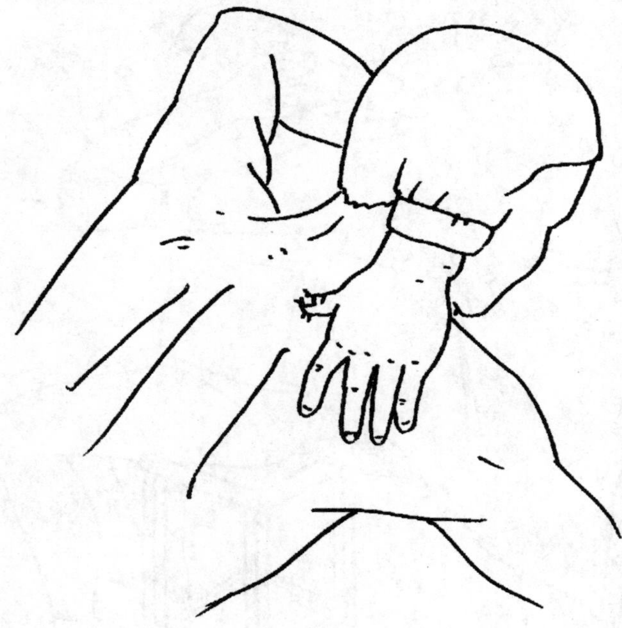

Finger stationary circular pressing technique on Quyuan (SI 13).

Manipulation

Place one thumb on Quyuan (SI 13) of the affected side while other four fingers on the back of the shoulder as shown in the picture. Knead Quyuan (SI 13) with the thumb for 3-5 minutes.

Points

Quyuan (SI 13): On the medial extremity of the suprascapular fossa, at the level of the spinous process of the second thoracic vertebra.

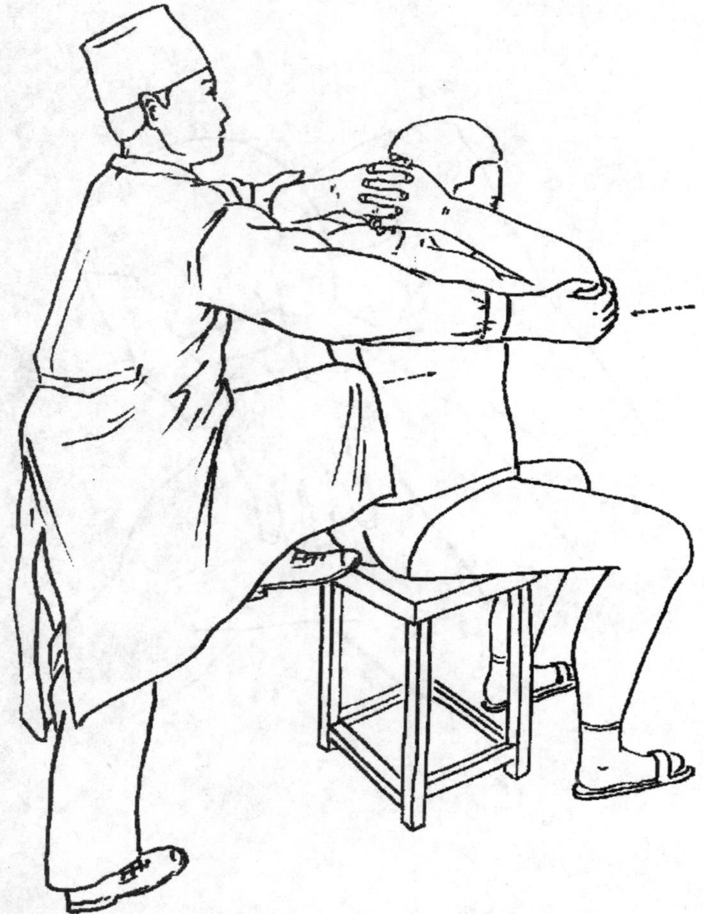

Chest stretching technique.

Manipulation

Let the hands go under the patient's armpits to the front, then wrap over and fix the patient's elbow regions. Place one knee on Taodao (GV 13) on patient's lower back. Instruct the patient to let his (her) chest stick out and take a deep breath. Slowly pull back the patient's elbows and let the knee push and press the back of the patient until the patient cannot inhale anymore. Repeat the manipulation 3-5 times.

Points

Taodao (GV 13): Below the spinous process of the first thoracic vertebra.

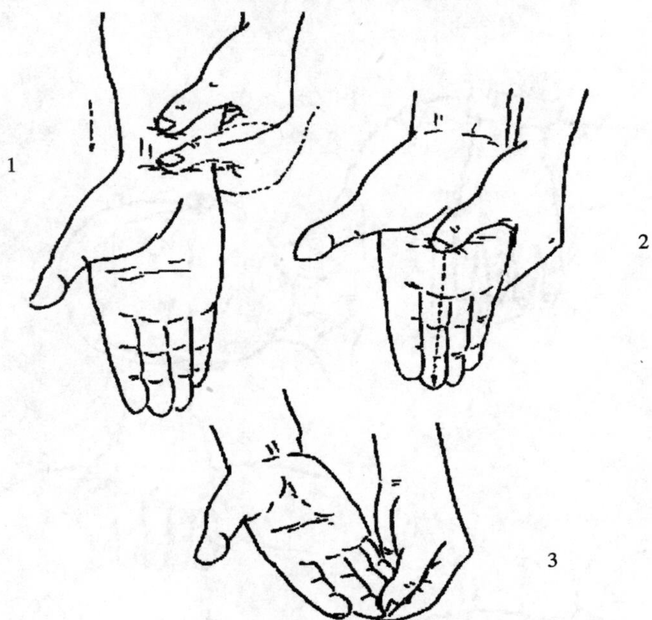

Opposite pressing technique on Waiguan (TE 5) and Neiguan (PC 6).

Manipulation

Place one thumb tip on Neiguan (PC 6) while other four fingertips on Waiguan (TE 5). Press the two acupoints for 1-2 minutes, then press and push downwards past Daling (PC 7) and Yangchi (TE 4) to Laogong (PC 8) and Zhongchong (PC 9). Rub each acupoint for 1-2 minutes. Repeat the manipulation for 1-3 times.

Points

1. Neiguan (PC 6): 2 *cun* above the transverse crease of the wrist, between the tendons of m. palmaris longus and m. flexor radialis.
2. Waiguan (TE 5): 2 *cun* above the transverse crease of the dorsum of wrist, between the radius and ulna.
3. Daling (PC 7): In the middle of the transverse crease of the wrist, between the tendons of m. palmaris longus and m. flexor carpi radialis.
4. Yangchi (TE 4): On the transverse crease of the dorsum of wrist, in the depression lateral to the tendon of m. extensor digitorum communis.
5. Laogong (PC 8): On the transverse crease of the palm, between the second and third metacarpal bones.
6. Zhongchong (PC 9): In the center of the tip of the middle finger.

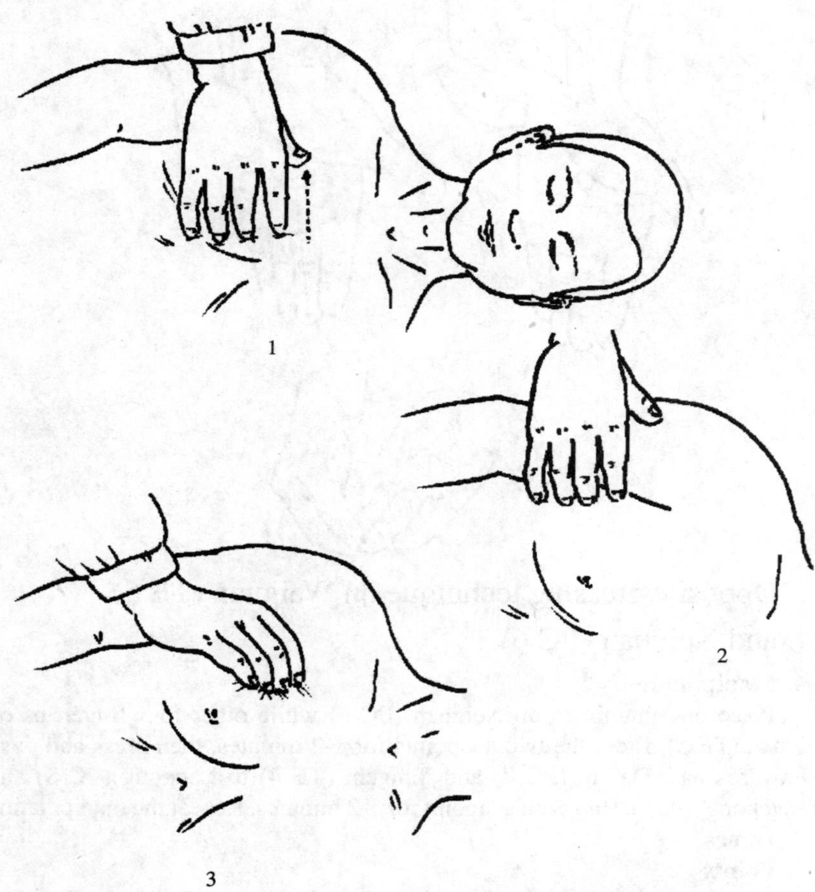

Pinching technique on the anterior of the axilla.

Manipulation

Place four finger-pulps at the medial border of musculus pectoralis major, rub transversely along the intercostal spaces to the front of the armpit for 1-2 minutes, then place a thumb under the armpit and other 4 fingers at the front of the armpit, repeatedly pinch and knead the lateral border of the pectoral muscle for 2-3 minutes.

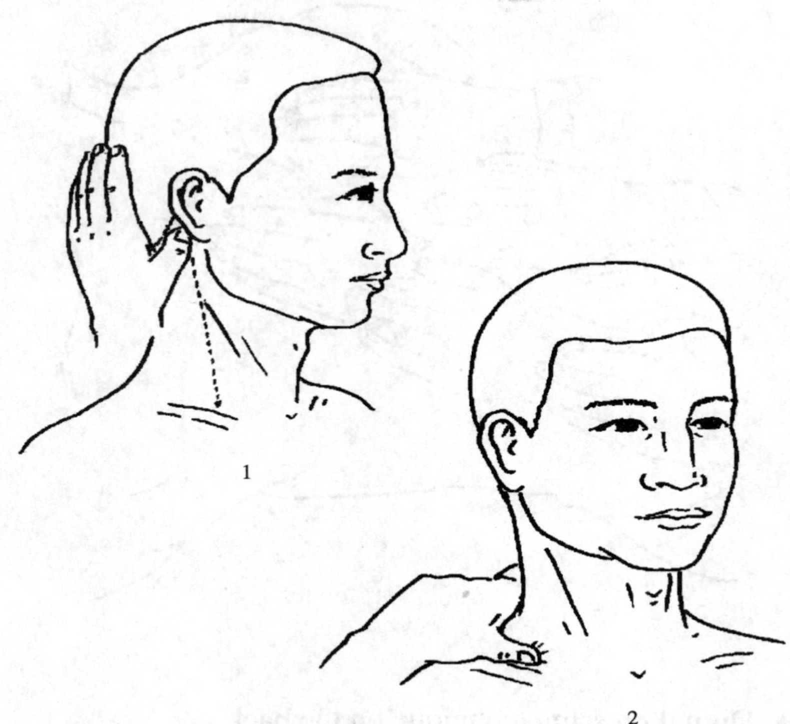

Pressing technique on Quepen (ST 12).

Manipulation

Place a thumb on Yifeng (TE 17), massage down to the neck in rubbing technique along the sternocleidomastoid muscle to Quepen (ST 12). Perform the manipulation 5-10 times. Then press Quepen (ST 12) 2-3 times, each time should last 15-30 seconds.

Points

1. Yifeng (TE 17): Posterior to the lobule of the ear, in the depression between the mandible and mastoid process.

2. Quepen (ST 12): In the midpoint of the supraclavicular fossa, 4 *cun* lateral to the anterior midline.

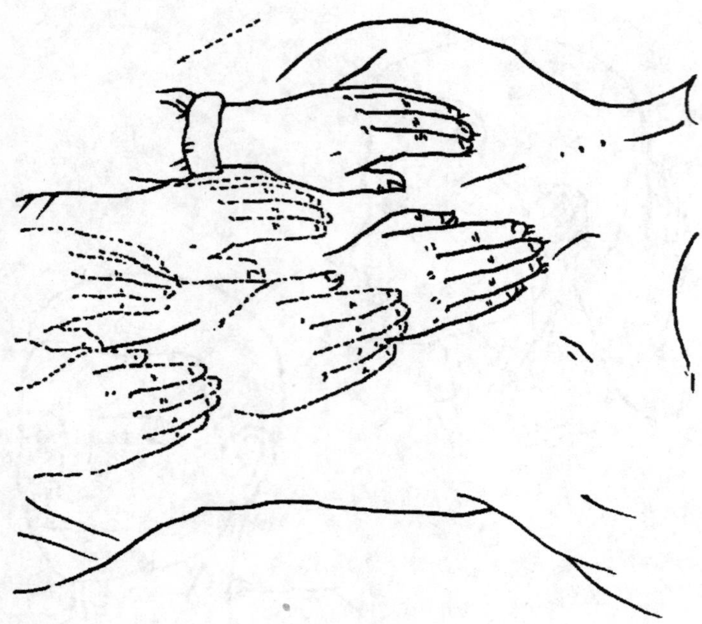

Digital pressing technique on the back.

Manipulation

Place four finger-pulps of both hands on Feishu (BL 13) and Pohu (BL 42), then slowly press the intercostal spaces in turn past Geshu (BL 17), Geguan (BL 46) and stop at Weishu (BL 21) and Weicang (BL 50). Repeat the manipulation for 3-5 times.

Points

1. Feishu (BL 13): At the level of the lower border of the spinous process of the third thoracic vertebra and 1.5 *cun* lateral to the posterior midline.
2. Pohu (BL 42): 1.5 *cun* lateral to Feishu (BL 13).
3. Geshu (BL 17): At the level of the lower border of the spinous process of the seventh thoracic vertebra and 1.5 *cun* lateral to the posterior midline.
4. Geguan (BL 46): 1.5 *cun* lateral to Geshu (BL 17).
5. Weishu (BL 21): At the level of the lower border of the spinous process of the twelfth thoracic vertebra and 1.5 *cun* lateral to the posterior midline.
6. Weicang (BL 50): 1.5 *cun* lateral to Weishu (BL 21).

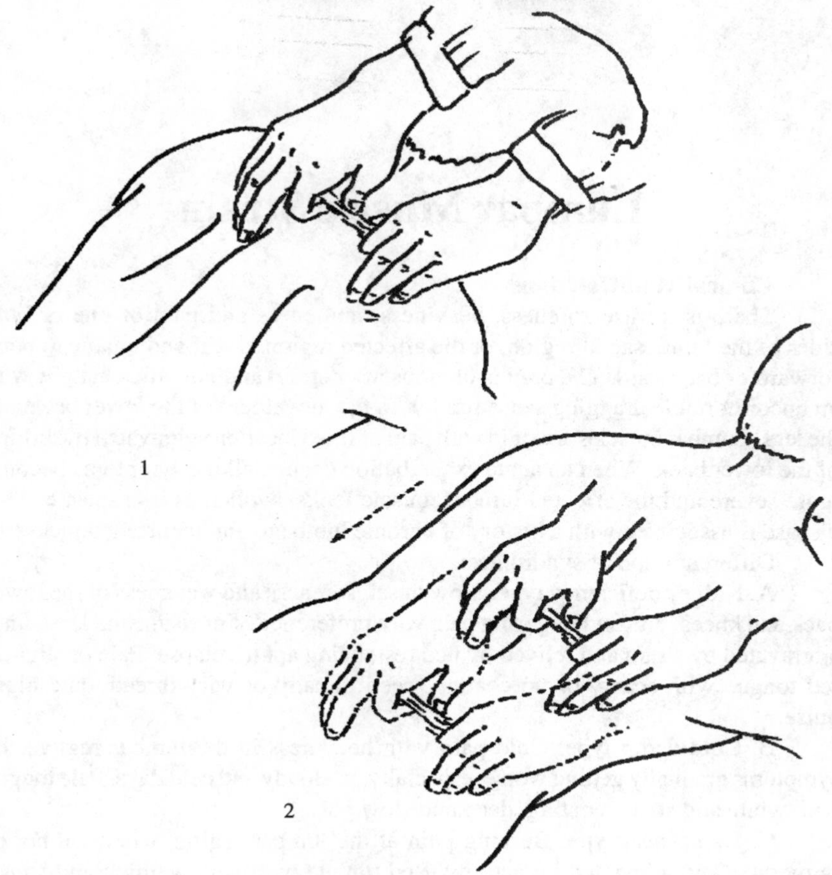

Holding and lifting techniques on the back.

Manipulation

Use two thumbs and index fingers to pinch Dazhu (BL 11) then keep on pinching and pulling up the muscle down the back past Pishu (BL 20) and stop at Guanyuanshu (BL 26). Repeat the manipulation for 3-5 times.

Points

1. Dazhu (BL 11): At the level of the lower border of the spinous process of the first thoracic vertebra and 1.5 *cun* lateral to the posterior midline.

2. Pishu (BL 20): At the level of the lower border of the spinous process of the eleventh thoracic vertebra and 1.5 *cun* lateral to the posterior midline.

3. Guanyuanshu (BL 26):At the level of the lower border of the spinous process of the fifth lumbar vertebra and 1.5 *cun* lateral to the posterior midline.

Lumbar Muscle Strain

Clinical Manifestations

There is diffuse soreness, heaviness, numbness and pain of one or both sides of the lumbosacral region, or the affected region is stiff and unable to bend forward or backward. The pain is obvious after strain and climatic changes with an uncomfortable dragging sensation felt in the movement of the lower back and the legs. Lumbar muscles are rigid with pain of fixed location aggravated by turning of the lower back. When an acute exacerbation occurs, all the symptoms become more severe and the affected lumbar muscle looks swollen as it is spastic. This disease is associated with a history of chronic lumbago and recurrent attacks.

Differentiation of syndromes:

A. Kidney deficiency type: Slow onset, soreness and weakness of the lower back and knees, dull and lingering pain with preference of pressure and kneading, aggravated by strain and relived by bed rest, being apt to relapse. Pale or slightly red tongue with scanty or no coating, deep thready or wiry thready and rapid pulse.

B. Cold-damp type: Cold pain with heaviness in the lumbar region, the symptoms gradually getting worse, especially on cloudy and cold days. Pale tongue with white and sticky coating, deep and slow pulse.

C. Damp-heat type: Burning pain at the lumbar region, worse on hot or rainy days and alleviated by activity. Red tongue with yellow, thick and sticky coating, soft rapid or wiry rapid pulse.

Treatment Principle

Warming and promoting *qi* and blood circulation, tonifying the kidney and strengthening the lumbus.

Tuina Techniques

A. Transverse rubbing technique on the lumbar region.
B. Straight rubbing technique on the lumbar region.
C. Stationary circular pressing technique on Yaoyan (EX-B7).
D. Overlapping palm pressing technique on the lumbar region.
E. Stepping technique on the back.
F. Stationary circular pressing technique on Weizhong (BL 40).

G. Pressing lumbus with leg pulling.

Addition or Subtraction Techniques

A. Kidney deficiency type:

Addition: Stationary circular pressing technique on Mingmen (GV 4).

B. Cold-damp type:

Addition: 1. Pushing technique on the back. 2. Heavy kneading technique on the posterior aspect of the leg.

C. Damp-heat type:

Addition: 1. Pushing technique on Dazhui (GV 14) and Yangguan (GV 3). 2. Stationary circular pressing technique on Sanyinjiao (SP 6). 3. Pushing technique on the lateral aspect of the foot. 4. Stationary circular pressing technique on Yongquan (KI 1).

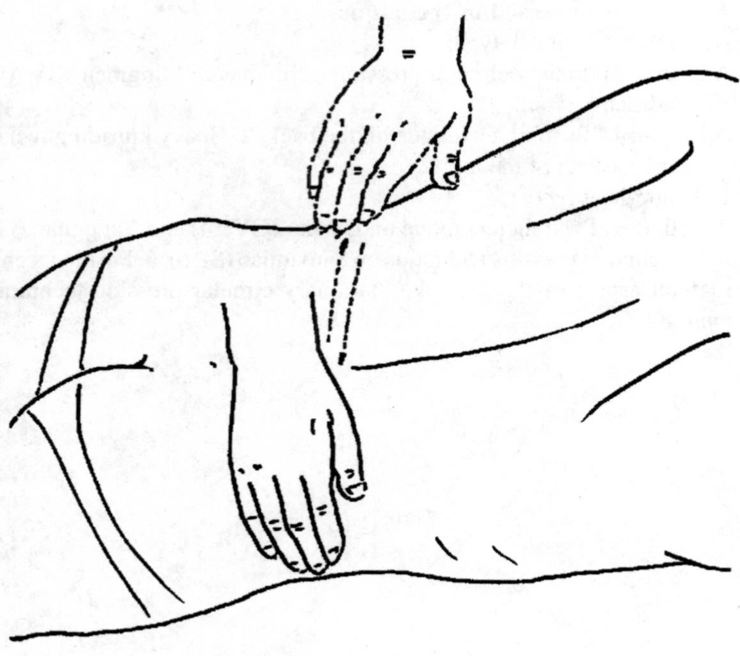

Transverse rubbing technique on the lumbar region.

Manipulation

Place a palm over unilateral Shenshu (BL 23), Qihaishu (BL 24) and Dachangshu (BL 25), rub to Daimai (GB 26), then rub back and forth between bilateral Daimai (GB 26). Repeat the massage 15-20 times.

Points

1. Shenshu (BL 23): At the level of the lower border of the spinous process of the second lumbar vertebra and 1.5 *cun* lateral to the midline.

2. Qihaishu (BL 24): At the level of the lower border of the spinous process of the third lumbar vertebra and 1.5 *cun* lateral to the midline.

3. Dachangshu (BL 25): At the level of the lower border of the spinous process of the fourth lumbar vertebra and 1.5 *cun* lateral to the midline.

4. Daimai (GB 26): Directly below the free end of the eleventh rib, at the level with the umbilicus.

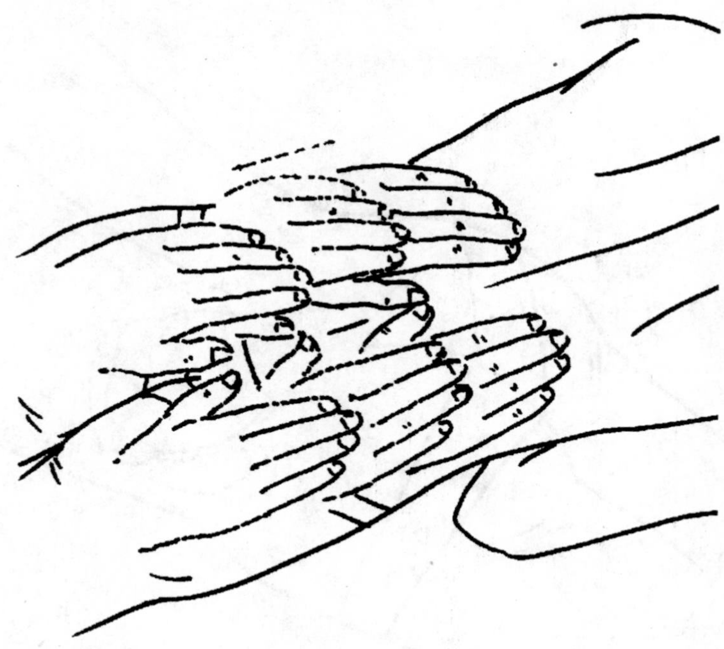

Straight rubbing technique on the lumbar region.

Manipulation

Place four finger-pulps of both hands on Weishu (BL 21) and Weicang (BL 50), massage straight downwards in rubbing method past Shenshu (BL 23), Zhishi (BL 52) and stop at Xiaochangshu (BL 27). Repeat the manipulation 5-15 minutes.

Points

1. Weishu (BL 21): At the level of the lower border of the spinous process of the twelfth thoracic vertebra and 1.5 *cun* lateral to the midline.
2. Weicang (BL 50): 1.5 *cun* lateral to Weishu (BL 21).
3. Shenshu (BL 23): At the level of the lower border of the spinous process of the second lumbar vertebra and 1.5 *cun* lateral to the midline.
4. Zhishi (BL 52): 1.5 *cun* lateral to Shenshu (BL 23).
5. Xiaochangshu (BL 27): At the level of the first posterior sacral foramen and 1.5 *cun* lateral to the midline.

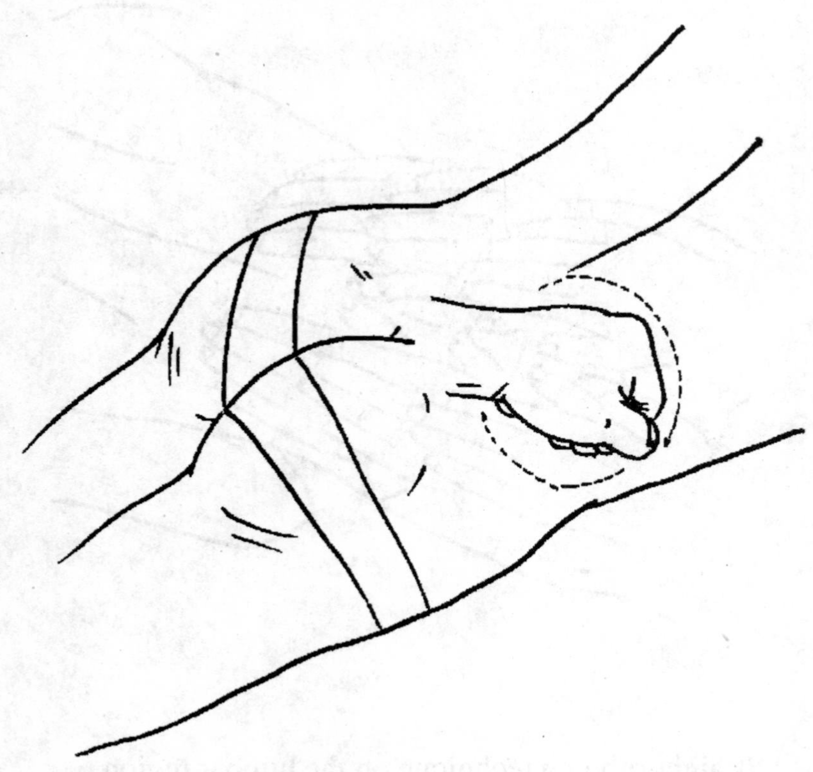

Stationary circular pressing technique on Yaoyan (Ex-B 7).

Manipulation

Make a partially clenched fist and use the back of the fist to knead Jingmen (GB 25) for 3-5 minutes.

Points

Jingmen (GB 25): On the lower border of the free end of the twelfth rib.

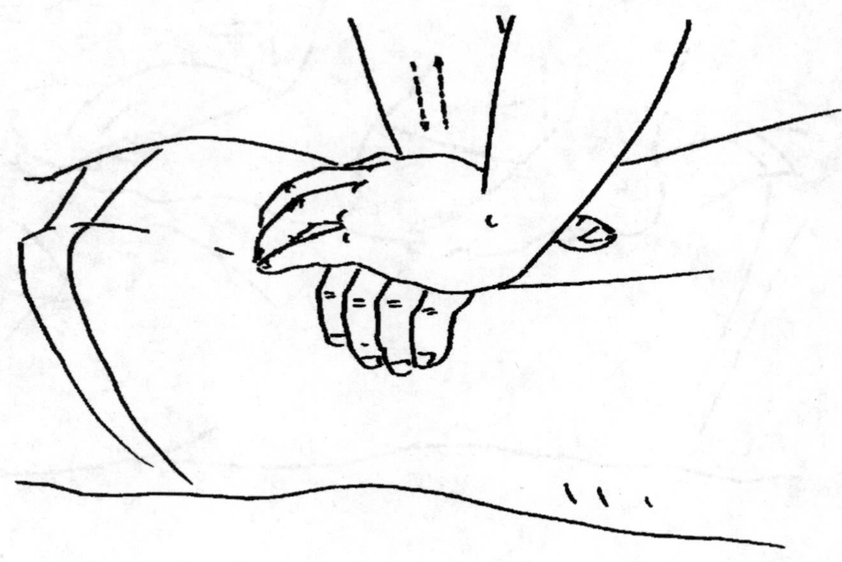

Overlapping palm pressing technique on the lumbar region.

Manipulation

Rub hands together until they are hot, then place one palm on Mingmen (GV 4) and place the other over it. Exert force and develop a rhythm while giving pressure on the acupoint 3-5 times.

Points

Mingmen (GV 4): Below the spinous process of the second lumbar vertebra.

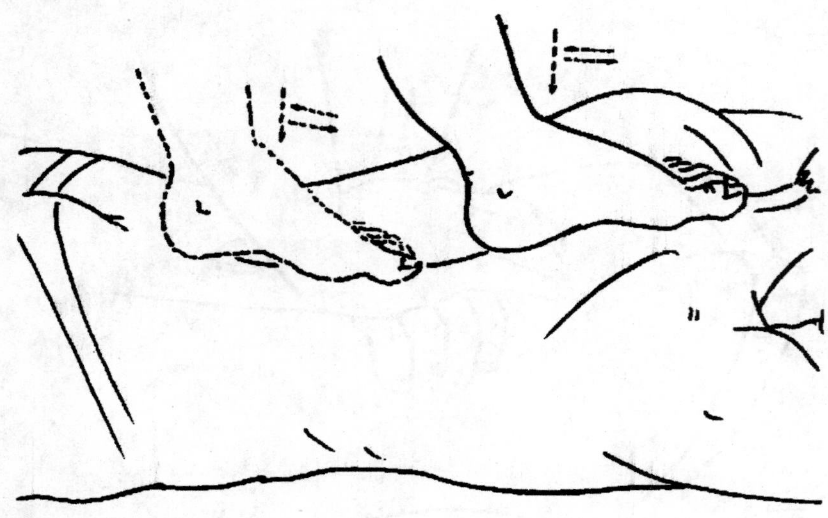

Stepping technique on the back.

Manipulation

Step by either foot on Dazhui (GV 14), Taodao (GV 13) and Shenzhu (GV 12), and then shake the foot to exert pressure to Baliao (BL 31—BL 34). Repeat the manipulation for 3-5 times.

Points

1. Dazhui (GV 14): Below the spinous process of the seventh cervical vertebra.
2. Taodao (GV 13): Below the spinous process of the first thoracic vertebra.
3. Shenzhu (GV 12): Below the spinous process of the third thoracic vertebra.
4. Baliao (BL 31—BL 34): In the first to fourth posterior sacral foramen of both sides.

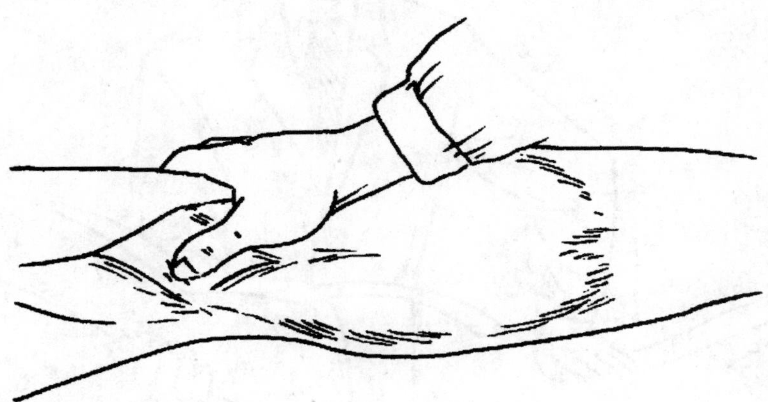

Stationary circular pressing technique on Weizhong (BL 40).

Manipulation

Place a thumb on Weizhong (BL 40) and vigorously press and knead the point for 3-5 minutes.

Points

Weizhong (BL 40): Midpoint of the transverse crease of the popliteal fossa.

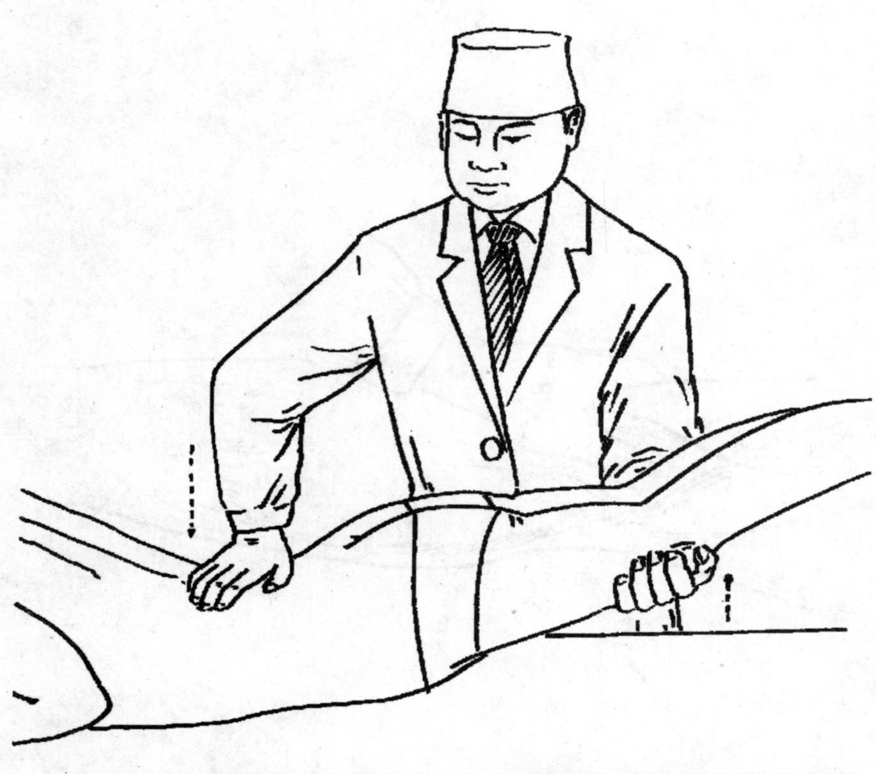

Pressing lumbus with leg pulling.

Manipulation

Place one palm on Yaoyangguan (GV 3) let the other hand grip both kneecaps. Apply pressure to the waist with the palm while lifting up the knees. Lift up the knees only as far as the patient can tolerate. Repeat the manipulation for 3-5 times.

Points

Yaoyangguan (GV 3): Below the spinous process of the fourth lumbar vertebra.

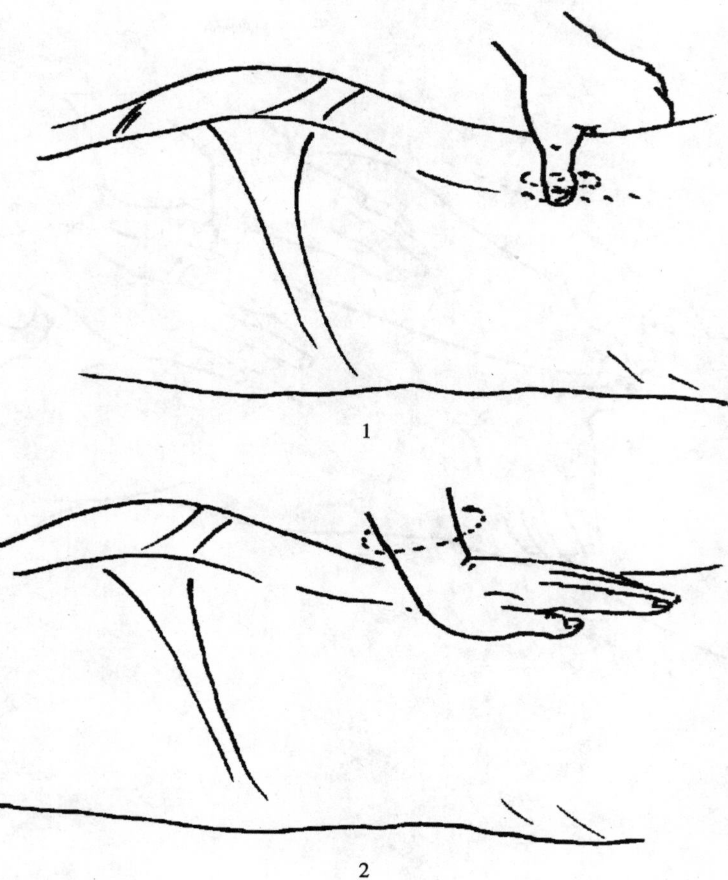

1

2

Stationary circular pressing technique on Mingmen (GV 4).

Manipulation

Place a thumb on Mingmen (GV 4) and press and knead the point for 2-3 minutes, then place the palm flat on the same area and conduct circular pressing for 1-2 minutes.

Points

Mingmen (GV 4): Below the spinous process of the second lumbar vertebra.

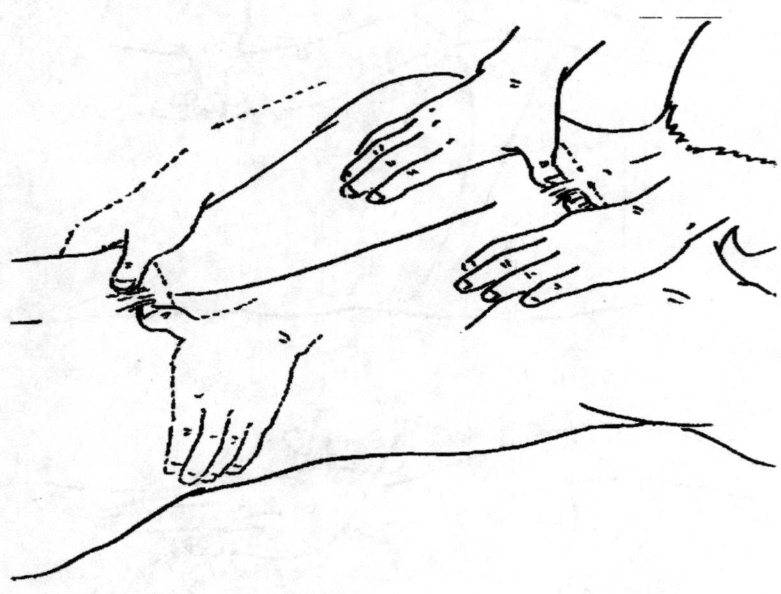

Pushing technique on the back.

Manipulation

Place two thumbs respectively on bilateral Dazhu (BL 11), squeeze and push straight downwards along both sides of the spine and stop at Dachangshu (BL 25). Repeat the manipulation for 3-5 times.

Points

1. Dazhu (BL 11): At the level of the lower border of the spinous process of the first thoracic vertebra and 1.5 *cun* lateral to the posterior midline.

2. Dachangshu (BL 25): At the level of the lower border of the spinous process of the fourth lumbar vertebra and 1.5 *cun* lateral to the posterior midline.

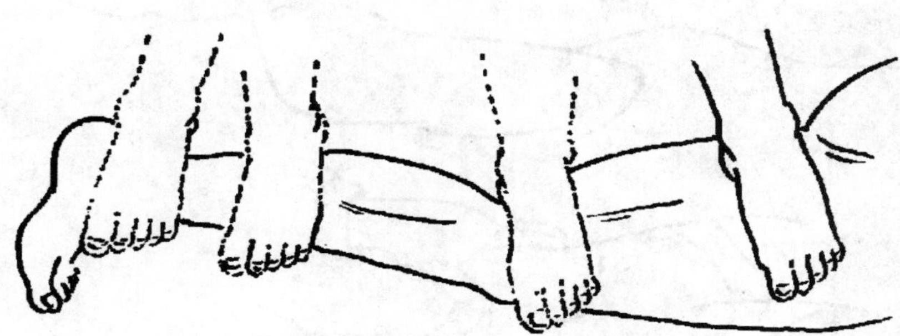

Heavy kneading technique on the posterior aspect of the leg.

Manipulation

Place a foot transversely on Chengfu (BL 36), then push and knead the leg downwards along the posterior midline of the leg past Weizhong (BL 40), Chengshan (BL 57) and stop at the ankle. Repeat the manipulation for 2-3 minutes.

Points

1. Chenfu (BL 36): In the middle of the transverse gluteal fold.
2. Weizhong (BL 40): Midpoint of the transverse crease of the popliteal fossa.
3. Chengshan (BL 57): In the top of the depression of the belly of m. gastrocnemius.

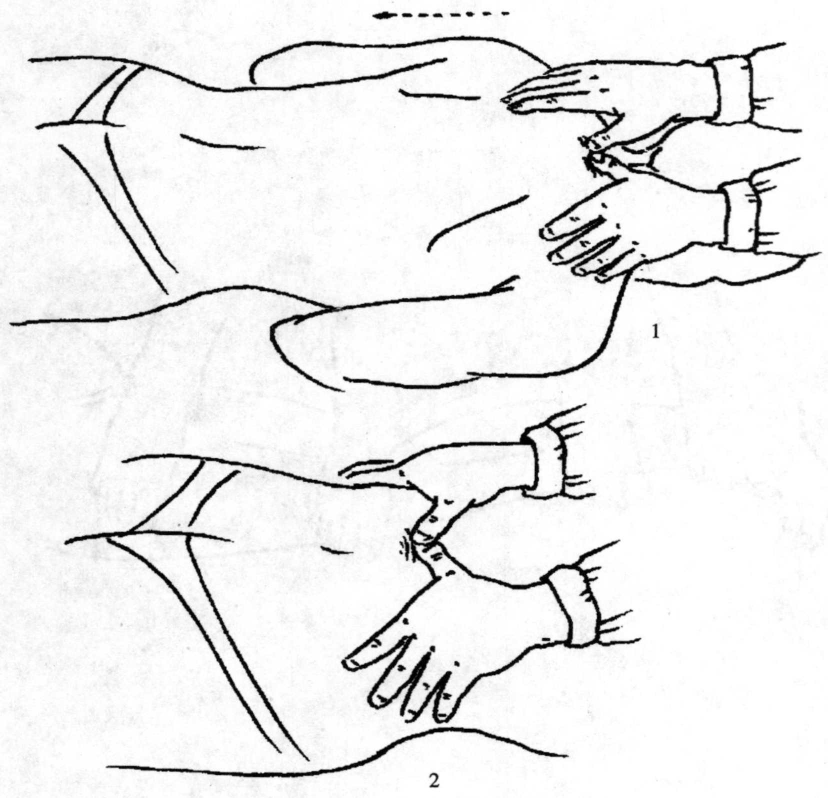

Pushing technique on Dazhui (GV 14) and Yangguan (GV 3).

Manipulation

Place two thumbs on Dazhui (GV 14), and knead the acupoint for 1-2 minutes, then push down along the spine (Governor Vessel) to Yaoyangguan (GV 3) and knead for 1-2 minutes. Repeat the manipulation for 2-3 times.

Points

1. Dazhui (GV 14): Below the spinous process of the seventh cervical vertebra.

2. Yaoyangguan (GV 3): Below the spinous process of the fourth lumbar vertebra.

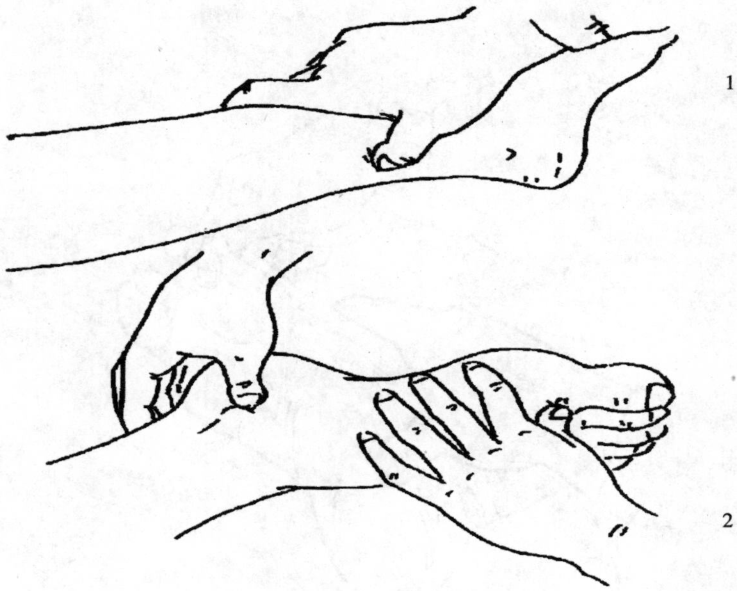

Stationary circular pressing technique on Sanyinjiao (SP 6).

Manipulation

Place a thumb tip on Sanyinjiao (SP 6), press and knead the acupoint for 3-5 minutes. Then move the thumb tip to Zhaohai (KI 6), meanwhile place the other thumb tip on Taichong (LR 3), press and knead the two acupoints at the same time for 1-3 minutes.

Points

1. Sanyinjiao (SP 6): 3 *cun* directly above the tip of the medial malleolus, on the posterior border of the medial aspect of the tibia.

2. Zhaohai (KI 6): In the depression of the lower border of the medial malleolus.

3. Taichong (LR 3): On the dorsum of the foot, in the depression distal to the junction of the first and second metatarsal bones.

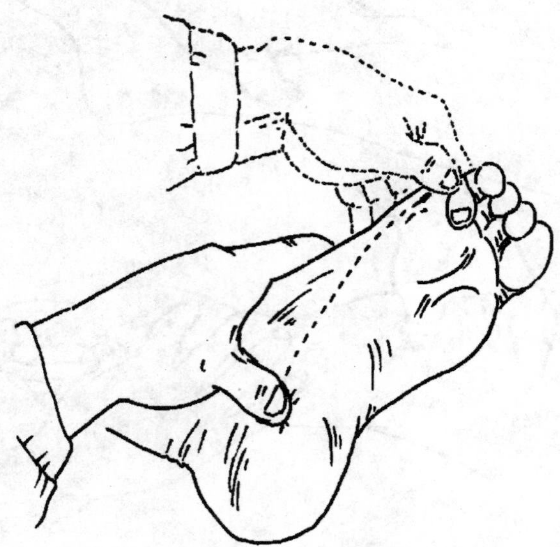

Pushing technique on the lateral aspect of the foot.

Manipulation

Place one thumb on Pucan (BL 61) while let other four fingers grip the back of the foot. Massage in pushing method with the thumb along the lateral margin of the foot (Bladder Meridian) to Zhiyin (BL 67), then press the distal section of the little toe to bend it down. Repeat the manipulation 2-5 minutes.

Points

1. Pucan (BL 61):Directly below the depression between the external malleolus and tendo calcaneus, at the junction of red and white skin.

2. Zhiyin (BL 67): On the lateral side of the small toe, about 0.1 *cun* posterior to the corner of the nail.

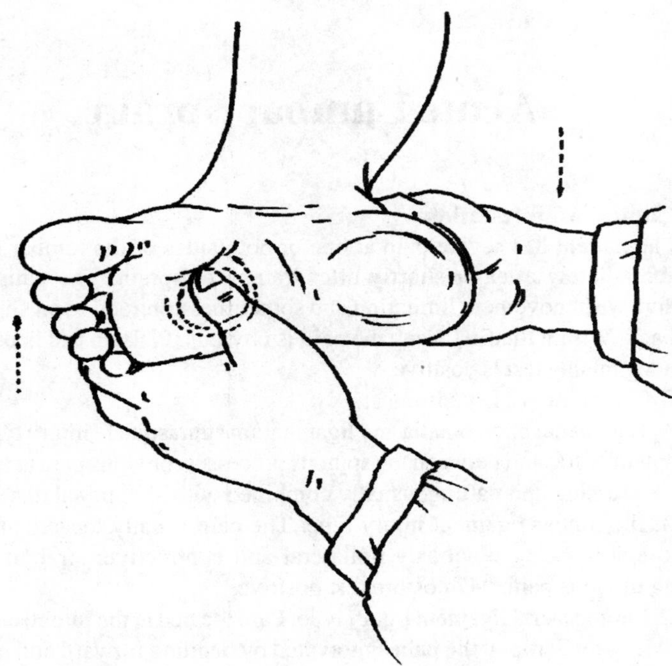

Stationary circular pressing technique on Yongquan (KI 1).

Manipulation

Use one hand to grab and press Achilles tendon and place the thumb of the other hand on Yongquan (KI 1) located at the bottom of the foot and knead the point clockwise and then counter-clockwise. Make 50 circles of kneading in each direction.

Points

Yongquan (KI 1): On the sole, in the depression when the foot is in plantar flexion, approximately at the junction of the anterior one third and posterior two thirds of the sole.

Acute Lumbar Sprain

Clinical Manifestations

The patient has severe pain at one or both sides of the lumbar region and back immediately after or shortly after trauma or sprain. The pain is mainly distending with movement limitation and sometimes contractive on slight turning of the back. Within the first week the pain is obvious. Pick-up test is positive and straight leg raising test is positive.

Differentiation of syndromes:

A. Ligamenta interspinalia and ligamentum supraspinale injury type: Painful point generally located between the spinous processes, obvious pain at the affected region in pressing and patting, usually combined with abdominal distention.

B. Iliolumbar ligament injury type: The pain usually located at the lower lumbar region, being obviously unilateral and contractive; straight leg rising inducing obvious pain, "4" posture test positive.

C. Lumbosacral ligament injury type: Pain located at the lumbosacral region with obvious tenderness, the pain aggravated by bending forward and radiating to the ipsilateral buttock, the thigh having distention and numbness.

Treatment Principle

Removing the obstruction from meridian and collateral, regulating *qi* and blood circulation, strengthening the lumbus and spine.

Tuina Techniques

A. Transverse rubbing technique on the lumbar region,
B. Straight rubbing technique on the lumbar region,
C. Lateral thumb pushing technique on the lumbar region.
D. Separate palm pushing technique on the lumbar region.
E. Pressing technique along the medial border of the iliac spine.
F. Opposite pressing and rubbing techniques on the side of the body.
G. Holding technique on the lumbar muscle.
H. Stationary circular pressing technique on Weizhong (BL 40).
I. Pressing lumbus with leg pulling.

Addition or Subtraction Techniques

A. Ligamenta interspinalia and ligamentum supraspinale injury type:

Addition: 1. Stationary circular pressing technique on Yaoyan (Ex-B 7). 2. Pushing and pressing the spinous process with lumbar rotation.

Subtraction: Separate palm pushing technique on the lumbar region.

B. Iliolumbar ligament injury type:

Addition: 1. Circular kneading technique on the sacro-iliac region. 2. Pressing technique along the superior border of the hip joint.

C. Lumbosacral ligament injury type:

Addition: 1. Kneading technique on the lumbosacral region. 2. Transverse rubbing technique on the sacrum. 3. Rotation technique of the lumbus.

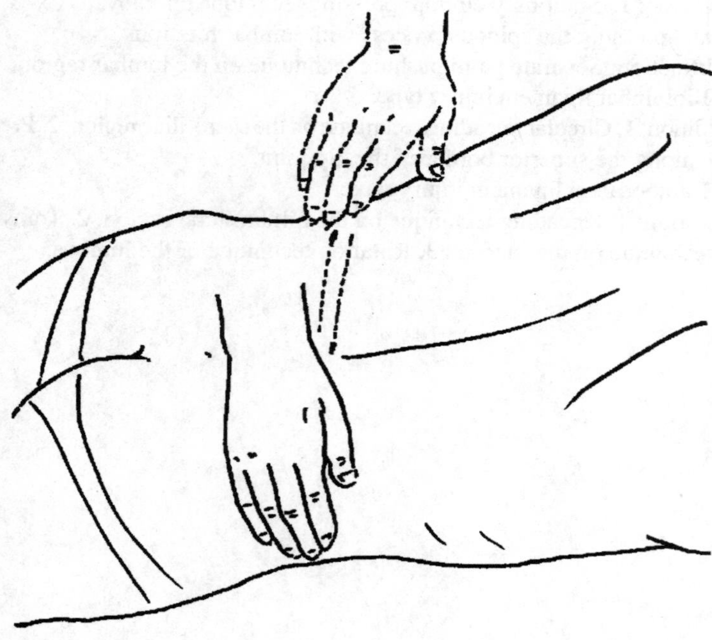

Transverse rubbing technique on the lumbar region.

Manipulation

Place a palm over unilateral Shenshu (BL 23), Qihaishu (BL 24) and Dachangshu (BL 25), rub to Daimai (GB 26), then rub back and forth between bilateral Daimai (GB 26). Repeat the massage 15-20 times.

Points

1. Shenshu (BL 23): At the level of the lower border of the spinous process of the second lumbar vertebra and 1.5 *cun* lateral to the midline.

2. Qihaishu (BL 24): At the level of the lower border of the spinous process of the third lumbar vertebra and 1.5 *cun* lateral to the midline.

3. Dachangshu (BL 25): At the level of the lower border of the spinous process of the fourth lumbar vertebra and 1.5 *cun* lateral to the midline.

4. Daimai (GB 26): Directly below the free end of the eleventh rib, at the level with the umbilicus.

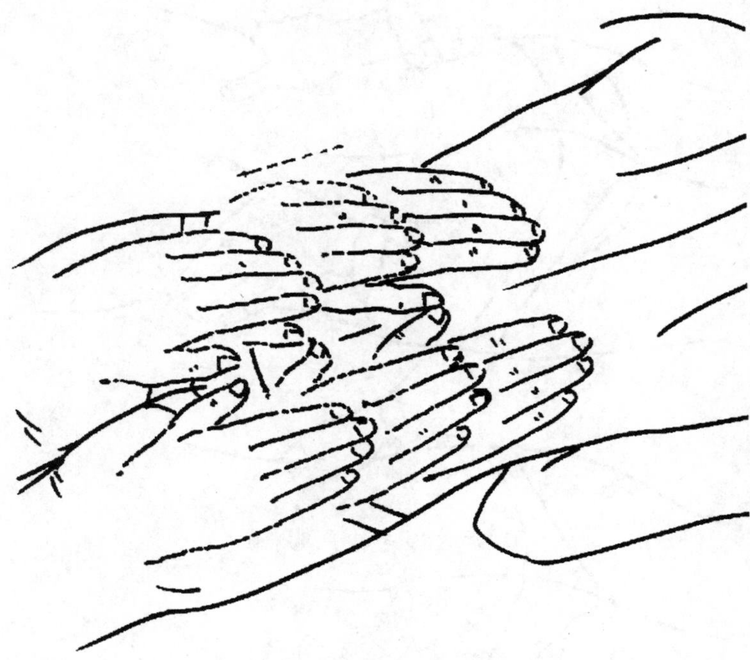

Straight rubbing technique on the lumbar region.

Manipulation

Place four finger-pulps of both hands on Weishu (BL 21) and Weicang (BL 50), massage straight downwards in rubbing method past Shenshu (BL 23), Zhishi (BL 52) and stop at Xiaochangshu (BL 27). Repeat the manipulation 5-15 minutes.

Points

1. Weishu (BL 21): At the level of the lower border of the spinous process of the twelfth thoracic vertebra and 1.5 *cun* lateral to the midline.

2. Weicang (BL 50): 1.5 *cun* lateral to Weishu (BL 21).

3. Shenshu (BL 23): At the level of the lower border of the spinous process of the second lumbar vertebra and 1.5 *cun* lateral to the midline.

4. Zhishi (BL 52): 1.5 *cun* lateral to Shenshu (BL 23).

5. Xiaochangshu (BL 27): At the level of the first posterior sacral foramen and 1.5 *cun* lateral to the midline.

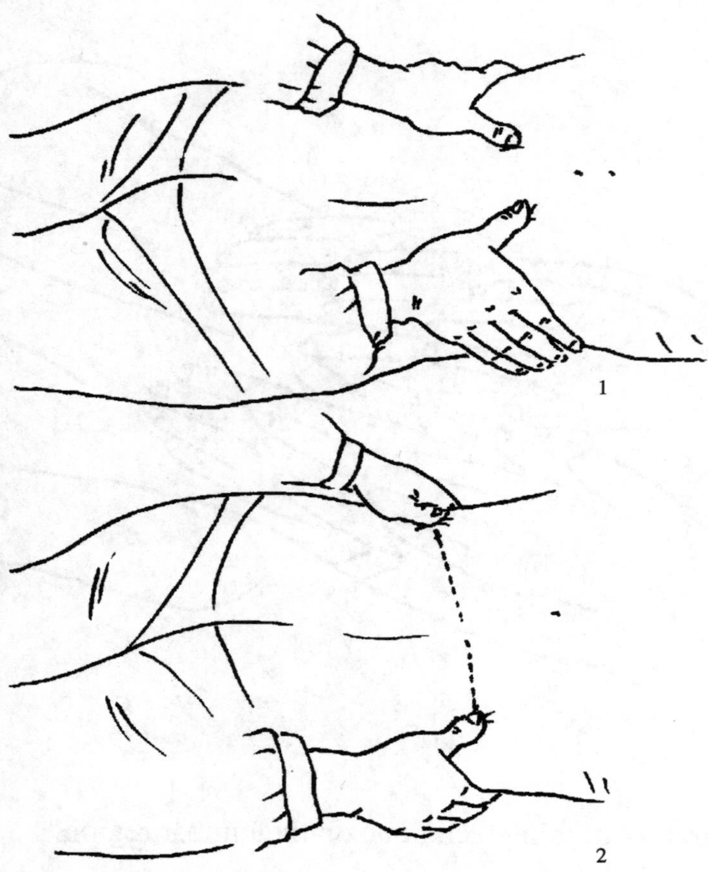

Lateral thumb pushing technique on the lumbar region.

Manipulation

Place two thumbs respectively on Shenshu (BL 23) and other four fingers around the waist. Then push laterally to the side of the back and stop at Daimai (GB 26). Repeat the manipulation for 1-3 minutes.

Points

1. Shenshu (BL 23): At the level of the lower border of the spinous process of the second lumbar vertebra and 1.5 *cun* lateral to the posterior midline.

2. Daimai (GB 26): Directly below the free end of the eleventh rib, at the level with the umbilicus.

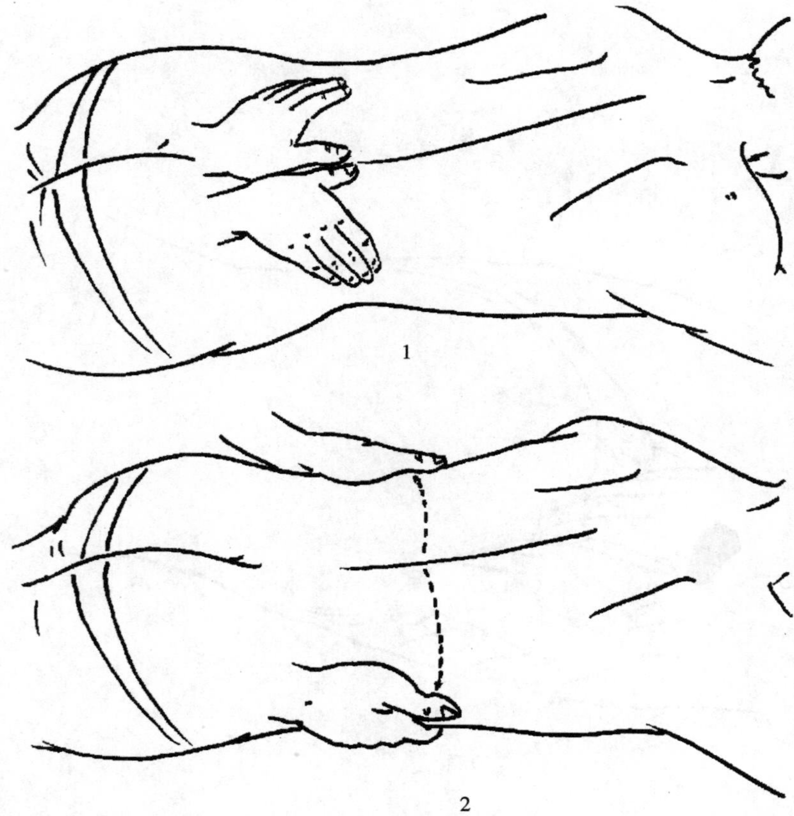

Separate palm pushing technique on the lumbar region.

Manipulation

Place the base of two palms on Mingmen (GV 4) as four fingers fan out covering both sides of the waist. Then push laterally past Shenshu (BL 23) to Daimai (GB 26). Repeat the manipulation for 3-5 minutes.

Points

1. Mingmen (GV 4): Below the spinous process of the second lumbar vertebra.

2. Shenshu (BL 23): At the level of the lower border of the spinous process of the second lumbar vertebra, 1.5 *cun* lateral to the posterior midline.

3. Daimai (GB 26): Directly below the free end of the eleventh rib, at the level with the umbilicus.

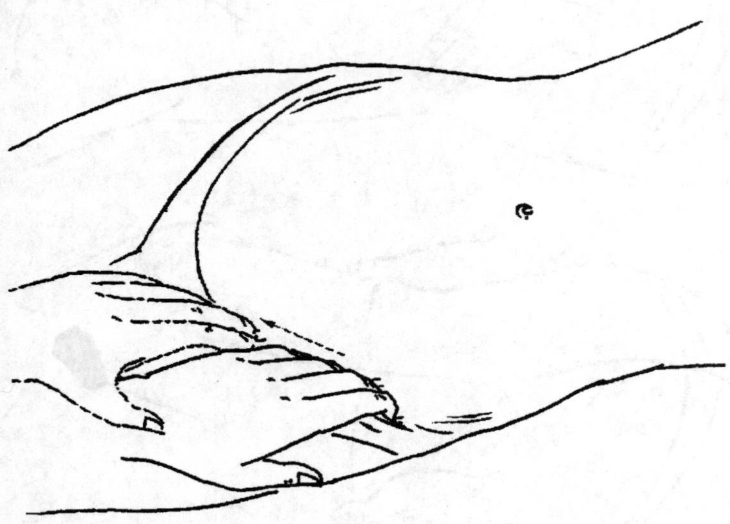

Pressing technique along the medial border of the iliac bone.

Manipulation

Place four fingertips on Wushu (GB 27) on the side of the ilium, then press and push down to Qichong (ST 30). Repeat the manipulation for 1-2 minutes.

Points

1. Wushu (GB 27): 0.5 *cun* anterior to the anterior superior iliac spine.

2. Qichong (ST 30): 5 *cun* directly below the center of the umbilicus and 2 *cun* lateral to the anterior midline.

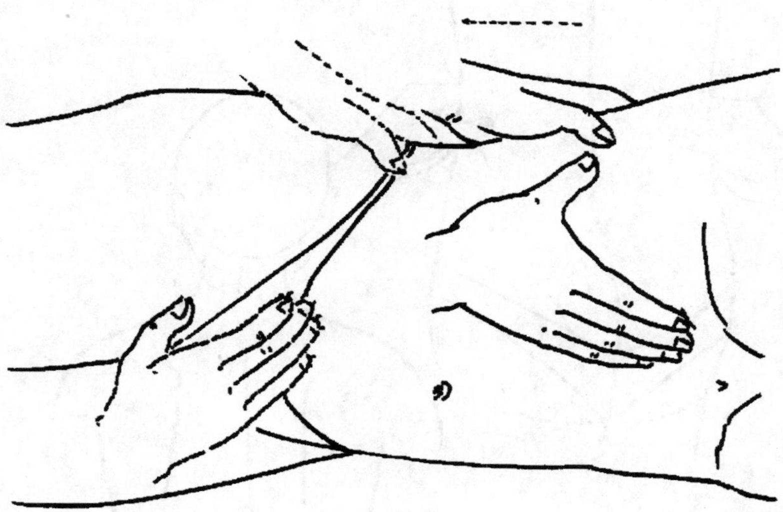

Opposite pressing and rubbing techniques on the side of the body.

Manipulation

Place four finger-pulps of both hands respectively over Burong (ST 19) located at the hypochondrium and Hunmen (BL 47) on the back, press the acupoints for 3-5 seconds, then rub downwards to Qichong (ST 30) and Yaoyan (Ex-B 7). Repeat the manipulation for 3-5 minutes.

Points

1. Burong (ST 19): 6 *cun* above the umbilicus and 2 *cun* lateral to the midline.

2. Hunmen (BL 47): At the level of the lower border of the spinous process of the ninth thoracic vertebra, 3 *cun* lateral to the posterior midline.

3. Qichong (ST 30): 5 *cun* directly below the center of the umbilicus and 2 *cun* lateral to the midline.

4. Yaoyan (Ex-B 7): At the level of the lower border of the spinous process of the fourth lumbar vertebra, in the depression 3-4 *cun* lateral to the midline.

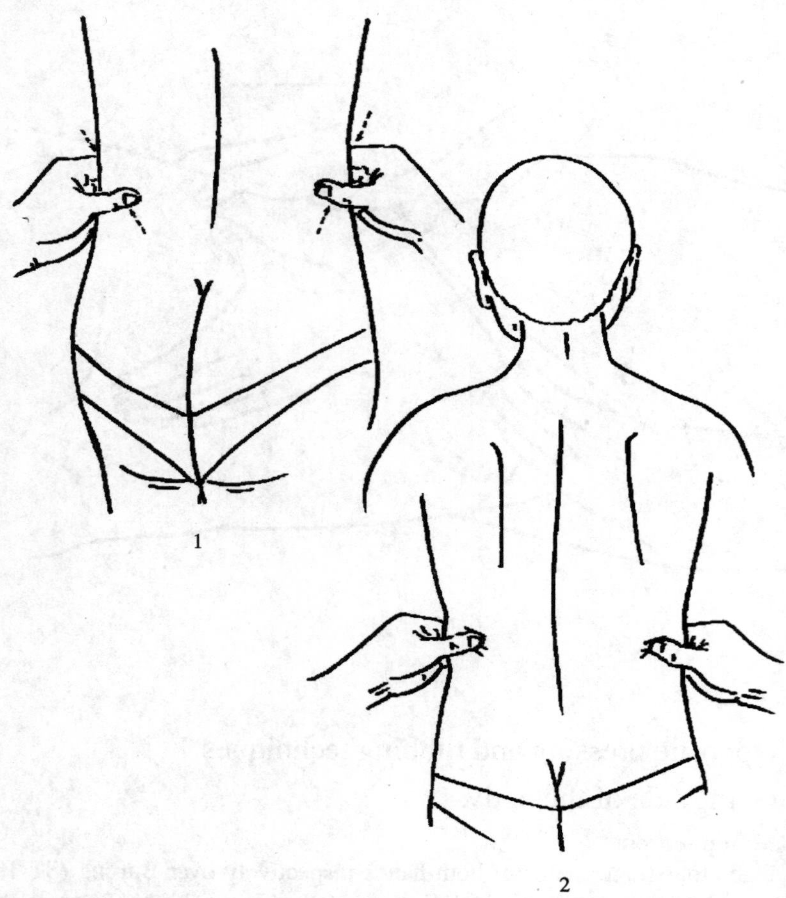

Holding technique on the lumbar muscle.

Manipulation

Place two thumbs respectively on Jingmen (GB 25), and other four fingers of both hands around Zhangmen (LR 13). Exert force and grab waist muscle to pull it 3-5 times, each time should last 2-3 seconds.

Points

1. Zhangmen (LR 13): At the free end of the eleventh floating rib.
2. Jingmen (GB 25): At the free end of the twelfth rib.

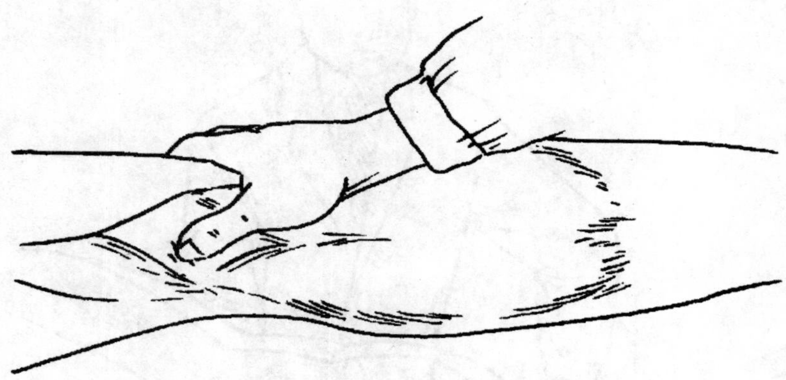

Stationary circular pressing technique on Weizhong (BL 40).

Manipulation

Place a thumb on Weizhong (BL 40) and vigorously press and knead the point for 3-5 minutes.

Points

Weizhong (BL 40): Midpoint of the transverse crease of the popliteal fossa.

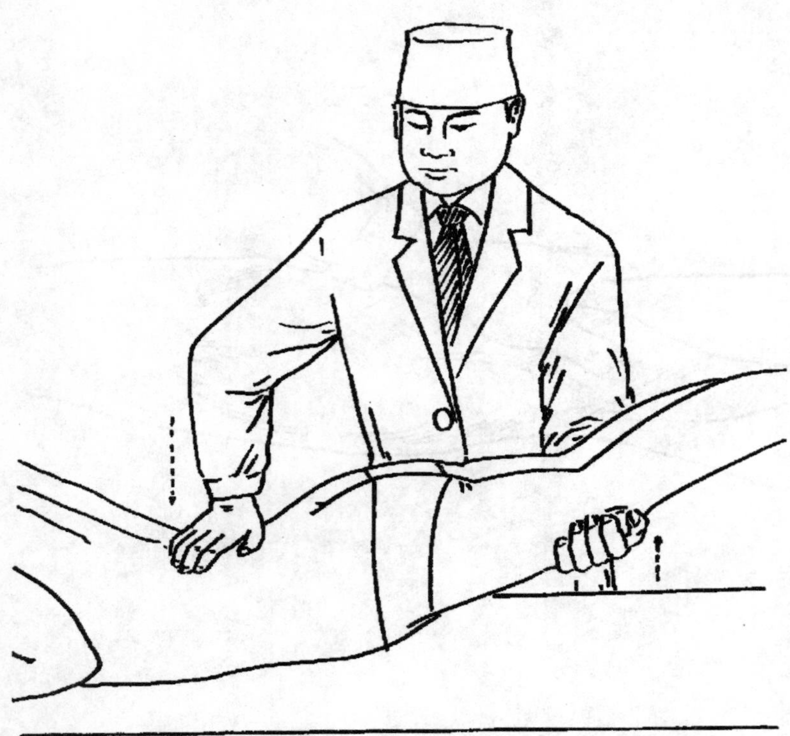

Pressing lumbus with leg pulling.

Manipulation

Place one palm on Yaoyangguan (GV 3) and let the other hand grip both kneecaps. Apply pressure to the waist with the palm while lifting up the knees. Lift up the knees only as far as the patient can tolerate. Repeat the manipulation for 3-5 times.

Points

Yaoyangguan (GV 3): Below the spinous process of the fourth lumbar vertebra.

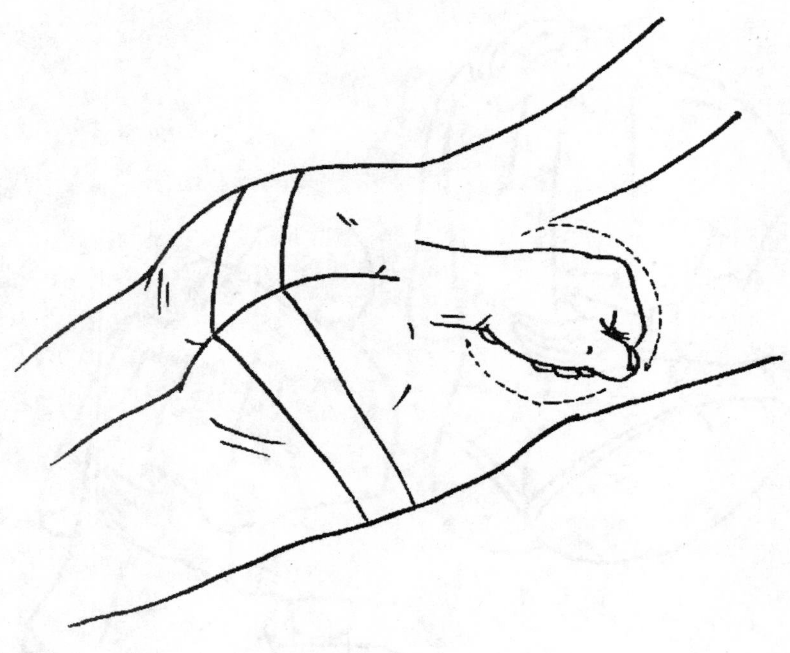

Stationary circular pressing technique on Yaoyan (Ex-B 7).

Manipulation

Place the back of a hollow fist on Jingmen (GB 25) and then knead circularly for 3-5 minutes.

Points

Jingmen (GB 25): On the lower border of the free end of the twelfth rib.

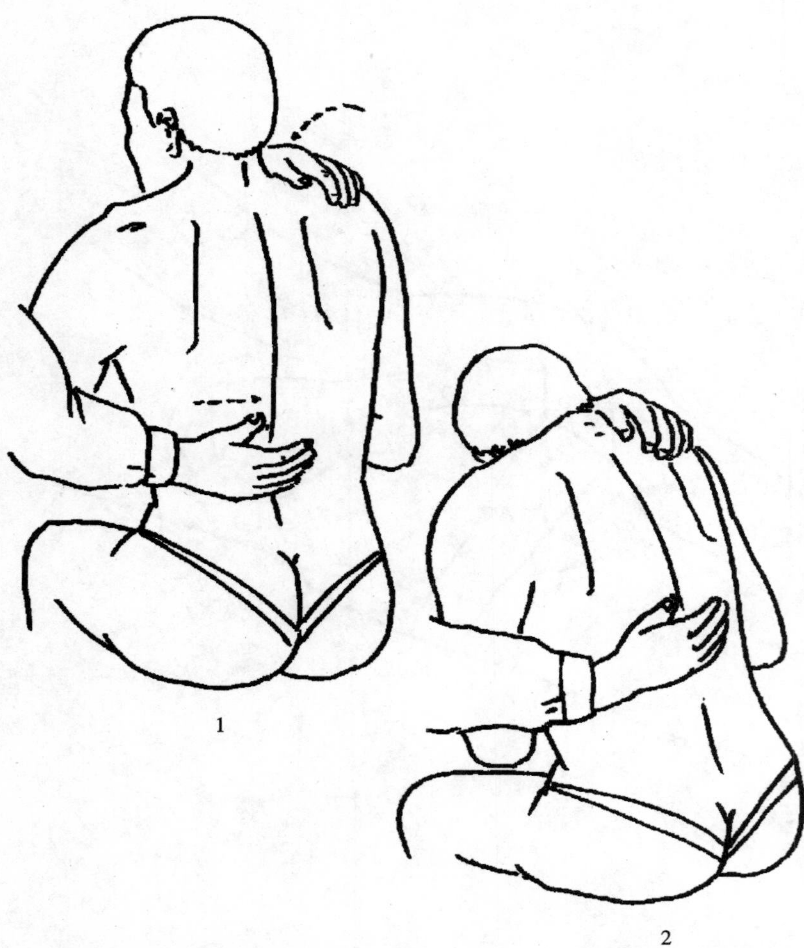

Pushing and pressing the spinous process while turning the lumbus.

Manipulation

Lay the forearm and palm on the shoulder of the patient to hold it still, then place the thumb of the other hand on the side of the affected spinous process. Pull the shoulder forward and downward to turn the lumbus. Meanwhile, let the thumb push and press the spinous process forcefully towards the opposite side for 30-60 seconds.

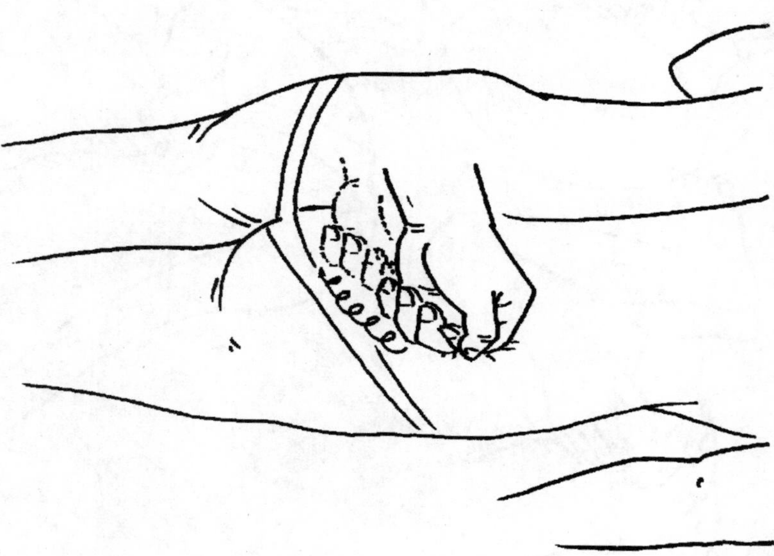

Circular kneading technique on the sacro-iliac region.

Manipulation

Place the back of a hollow fist on Baohuang (BL 53), conduct kneading in a slight diagonal direction towards the buttock middle and stop at Baihuanshu (BL 30). Repeat the fist kneading for 3-5 minutes.

Points

1. Baohuang (BL 53): At the level of the second sacral posterior foramen and 3 *cun* lateral to the midline.

2. Baihuanshu (BL 30): At the level of the fourth sacral posterior foramen and 1.5 *cun* lateral to the midline.

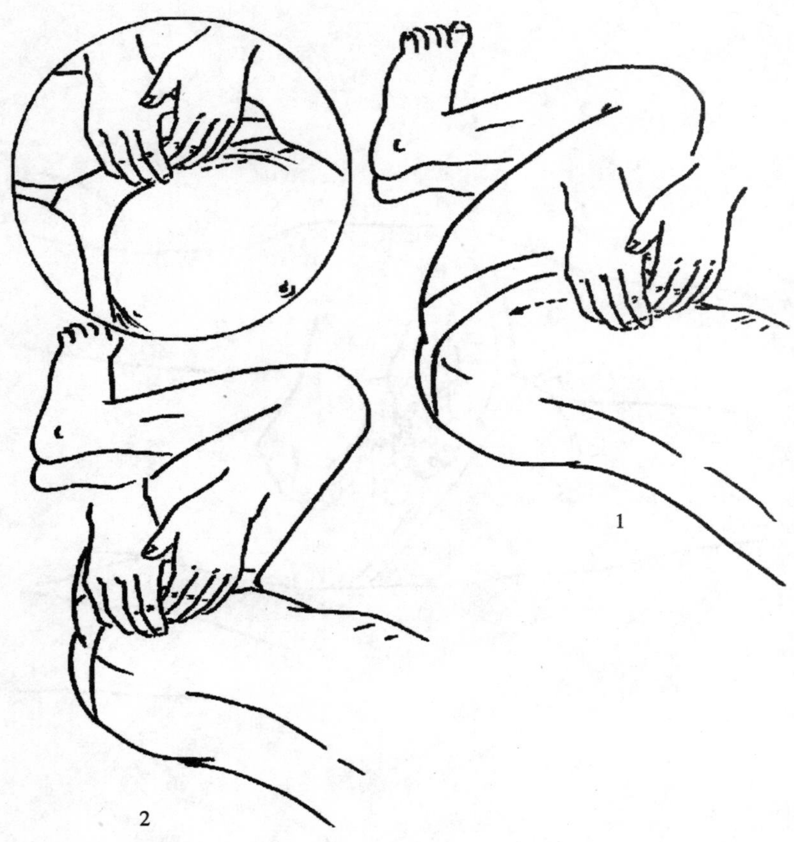

Pressing technique along the superior border of the hip joint.

Manipulation

Place four finger-pulps of both hands on Wushu (GB 27) and Weidao (GB 28), then press along the iliac spine and stop at Baohuang (BL 53). Repeat the manipulation for 1-3 minutes.

Points

1. Wushu (GB 27): 1.5 *cun* anterior to the anterior superior iliac spine.
2. Weidao (GB 28): 0.5 *cun* anterior and inferior of Wushu (GB 27).
3. Baohuang (BL 53): At the level of the second sacral posterior foramen and 3 *cun* lateral to the midline.

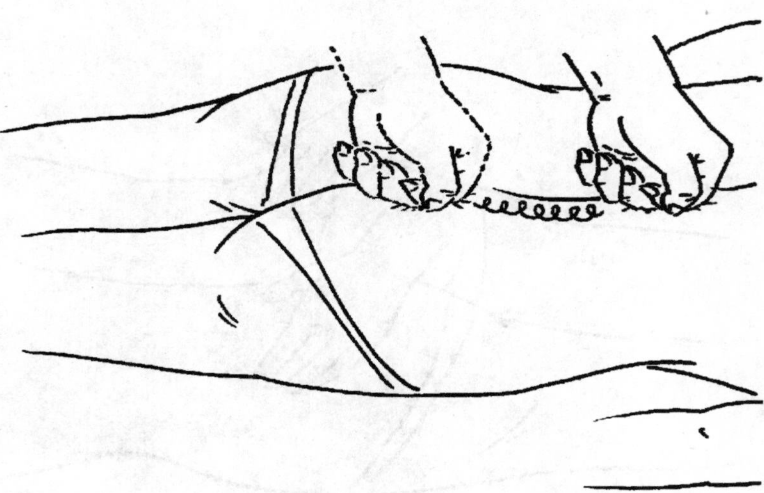

Kneading technique on the lumbosacral region.

Manipulation

Place the back of partially clenched fist on Mingmen (GV 4) and Shenshu (BL 23), then perform kneading technique down the spine to Yaoshu (GV 2) and Baihuanshu (BL 30). Repeat the manipulation for 2-5 minutes.

Points

1. Mingmen (GV 4): Below the spinous process of the second lumbar vertebra.

2. Shenshu (BL 23): At the level of the lower border of the spinous process of the second lumbar vertebra, 1.5 *cun* lateral to the midline.

3. Yaoshu (GV 2): In the hiatus of the sacrum.

4. Baihuanshu (BL 30): At the level of the fourth posterior sacral foramen, 1.5 *cun* lateral to the midline.

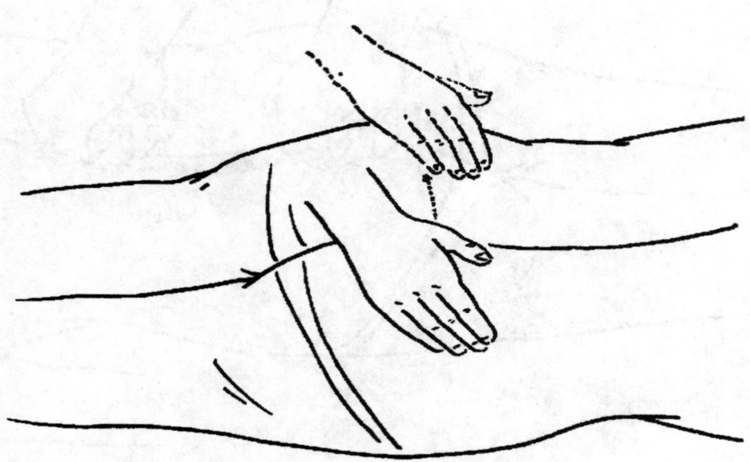

Transverse rubbing technique on the sacrum.

Manipulation

Place one palm on unilateral Baohuang (BL 53), then rub transversely past Baliao (BL 31—BL 34) and stop at Baohuang (BL 53) on the opposite side. Repeat the manipulation for 3-5 minutes.

Points

1. Baohuang (BL 53): At the level of the second sacral posterior foramen and 3 *cun* lateral to the midline.

2. Baliao (BL 31—BL 34): In the first to fourth posterior sacral foramen of both sides.

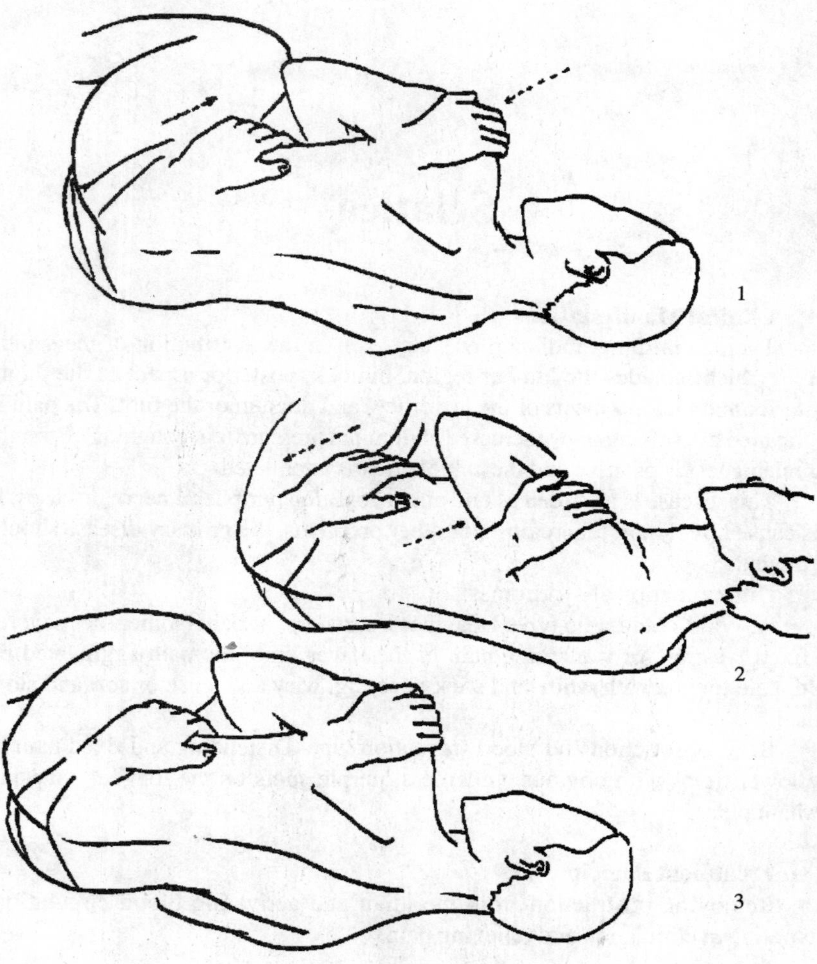

Rotation technique of the lumbus.

Manipulation

Place one hand over the shoulder while let the other hand grab the hip (on the same side of the shoulder), then use the hands to move the patient back and forth slightly to relax waist muscle. Then suddenly push the shoulder forward and pull the hip back, then vice-versa. Do it once on each side.

Sciatica

Clinical Manifestations

There is burning, radiating or sharp pain in the distribution of the sciatic nerve, which includes the lumbar region, buttock, posterior aspect of the thigh, posterior and lateral aspects of the lower leg, and dorsum of the foot. The pain is aggravated by walking or by increased abdominal pressure (eg. coughing). Straight leg raising test is positive and the ankle reflex is attenuated.

This disease is regarded as one of the common peripheral nerve diseases. If it is caused by tumor, tuberculosis or other problems, the primary disease should be treated.

Differentiation of syndromes:

A. Wind-cold-damp type: Heaviness, soreness, or pain (sometimes severe) of fixed location, or wandering pain in the lower limb; the pain aggravated by cold, pale tongue with white and sticky coating, wiry and tense or soft and slow pulse.

B. *Qi* obstruction and blood stagnation type: Distending and fixed pain in the lower limbs with obvious tenderness, purple spots on the tongue, wiry and hesitant pulse.

Treatment Principle

Removing obstruction from meridian and activating blood circulation, promoting *qi* circulation and relieving pain.

Tuina Techniques

A. Straight rubbing technique on the lumbar region.
B. Stationary circular pressing technique on Mingmen (GV 4)
C. Pushing technique on the posterior aspect of the leg.
D. Heavy kneading technique on the posterior aspect of the leg.
E. Pressing technique on the lower leg.
F. Pushing technique on the lateral aspect of the foot.
G. Extension and flexion technique of the ankle.
H. Rotation technique of the big toe.

Addition or Subtraction Techniques

A. Wind-cold-damp type:

Addition: 1. Pushing technique on Dazhui (GV 14) and Yangguan (GV 3). 2. Pushing technique on the buttock. 3. Pressing technique on Huantiao (GB 30).

B. *Qi* obstruction and blood stagnation type:

Addition: 1. Lateral thumb pushing technique on the lumbar region. 2. Straight pushing technique on the lumbar region for reinforcing *qi*. 3. Stationary circular pressing technique on Weizhong (BL 40). 4. Pressing technique along the middle line of the abdomen.

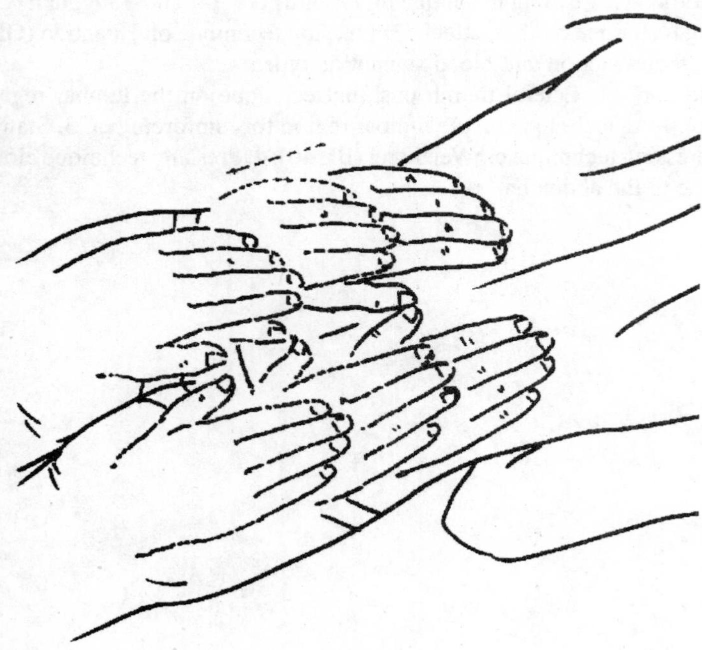

Straight rubbing technique on the lumbar region.

Manipulation

Place four finger-pulps of both hands on Weishu (BL 21) and Weicang (BL 50), massage straight downwards in rubbing method past Shenshu (BL 23), Zhishi (BL 52) and stop at Xiaochangshu (BL 27). Repeat the manipulation 5-15 minutes.

Points

1. Weishu (BL 21): At the level of the lower border of the spinous process of the twelfth thoracic vertebra and 1.5 *cun* lateral to the midline.

2. Weicang (BL 50): 1.5 *cun* lateral to Weishu (BL 21).

3. Shenshu (BL 23): At the level of the lower border of the spinous process of the second lumbar vertebra and 1.5 *cun* lateral to the midline.

4. Zhishi (BL 52): 1.5 *cun* lateral to Shenshu (BL 23).

5. Xiaochangshu (BL 27): At the level of the first posterior sacral foramen and 1.5 *cun* lateral to the midline.

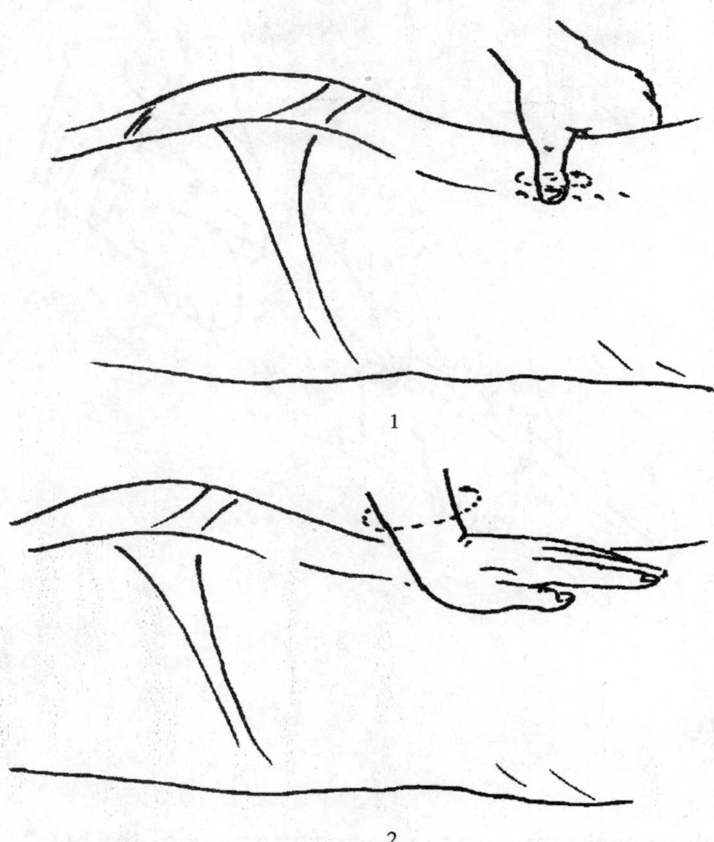

Stationary circular pressing technique on Mingmen (GV 4).

Manipulation

Place a thumb on Mingmen (GV 4), knead and press the point for 2-3 minutes, then place the palm flat on the same area and press for 1-2 minutes.

Points

Mingmen (GV 4): Below the spinous process of the second lumbar vertebra.

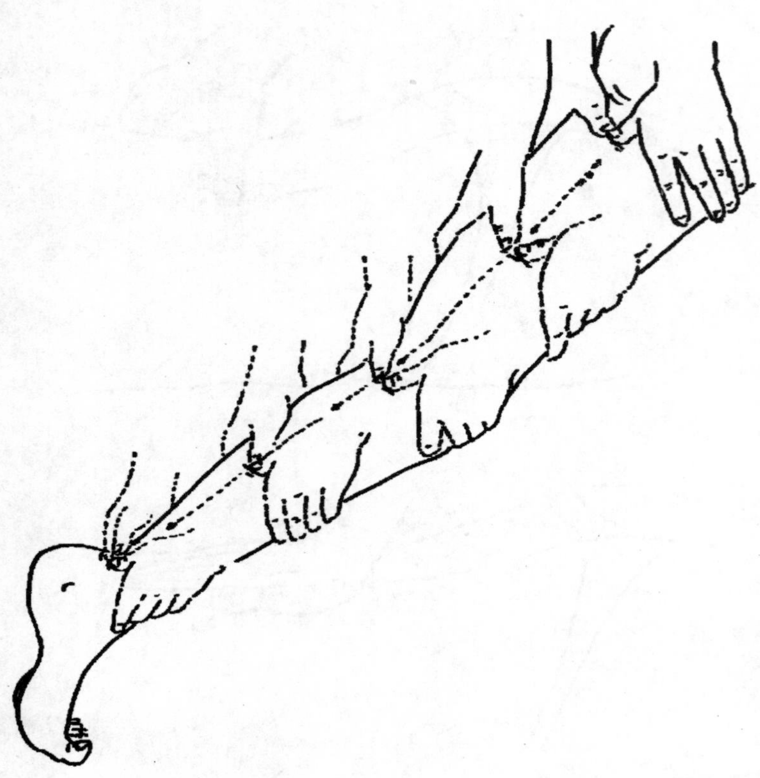

Pushing technique on the posterior aspect of the leg.

Manipulation

Place two thumbs on Chengfu (BL 36) and other fingers around both sides of the leg, then press and push downwards past Yinmen (BL 37), Weizhong (BL 40), Chengshan (BL 57) and stop at the ankle. Repeat the manipulation for 3-5 minutes.

Points

1. Chengfu (BL 36): In the middle of the transverse gluteal fold.
2. Yinmen (BL 37): 6 *cun* directly below Chengfu (BL 36).
3. Weizhong (BL 40): Midpoint of the transverse crease of the popliteal fossa.
4. Chengshan (BL 57): In the top of the depression of the belly of m. gastrocnemius.

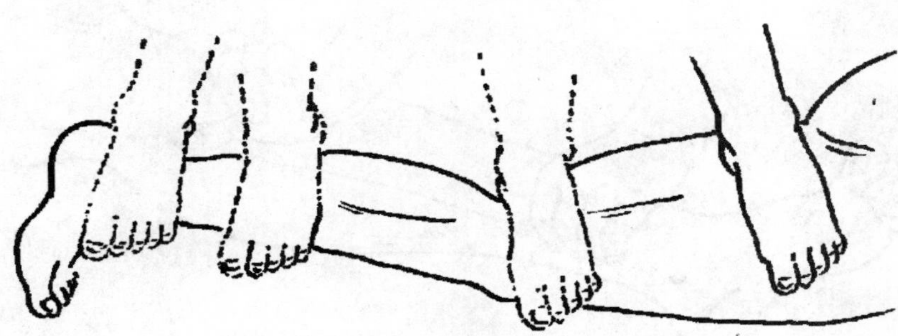

Heavy kneading technique on the posterior aspect of the leg.

Manipulation

Place the bottom of foot on Chengfu (BL 36) transversely, then push and knead downwards along the posterior midline of the leg past Weizhong (BL 40), Chengshan (BL 57) and stop at the ankle. Repeat the manipulation for 2-3 minutes.

Points

1. Chenfu (BL 36): In the middle of the transverse gluteal fold.
2. Weizhong (BL 40): Midpoint of the transverse crease of the popliteal fossa.
3. Chengshan (BL 57): In the top of the depression of the belly of m. gastrocnemius.

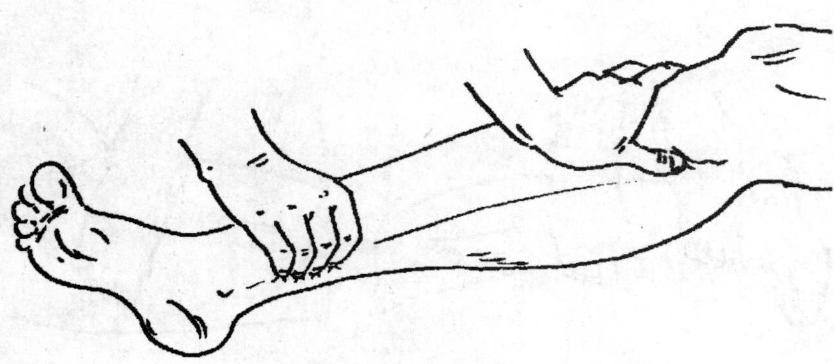

Pressing technique on the lower leg.

Manipulation

Place one thumb on Yinlingquan (SP 9) and the other four fingers on the side of the leg. Place the four fingertips of other hand on Sanyinjiao (SP 6) and lougu (SP 7). Press the points simultaneously 3-5 times, each time should last 15-30 seconds.

Points

1. Yinlingquan (SP 9): On the lower border of the medial condyle of the tibia, in the depression on the medial border of the tibia.

2. Sanyinjiao (SP 6): 3 *cun* directly above the tip of the medial malleolus, on the posterior border of the medial aspect of the tibia.

3. Lougu (SP 7): 3 *cun* directly above Sanyinjiao (SP 6).

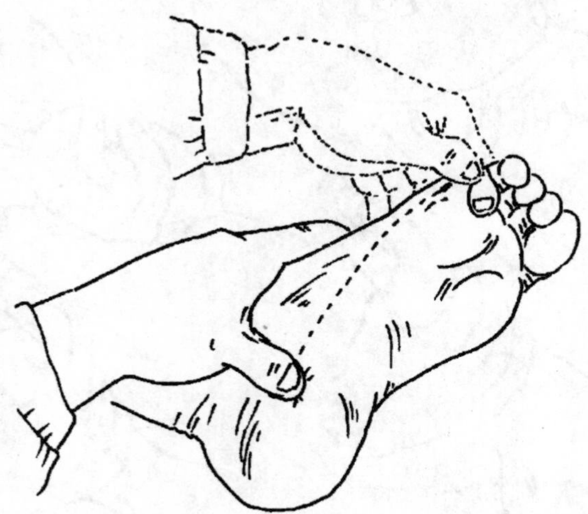

Pushing technique on the lateral aspect of the foot.

Manipulation

Place one thumb on Pucan (BL 61) and grip the back of the foot with other four finger. Push along the lateral margin of the foot (Bladder Meridian) to Zhiyin (BL 67), then Press the distal section of the little toe to bend it down. Repeat the manipulation 2-5 minutes.

Points

1. Pucan (BL 61):Directly below the depression between the external malleolus and tendo calcaneus, at the junction of red and white skin.

2. Zhiyin (BL 67): On the lateral side of the small toe, about 0.1 *cun* posterior to the corner of the nail.

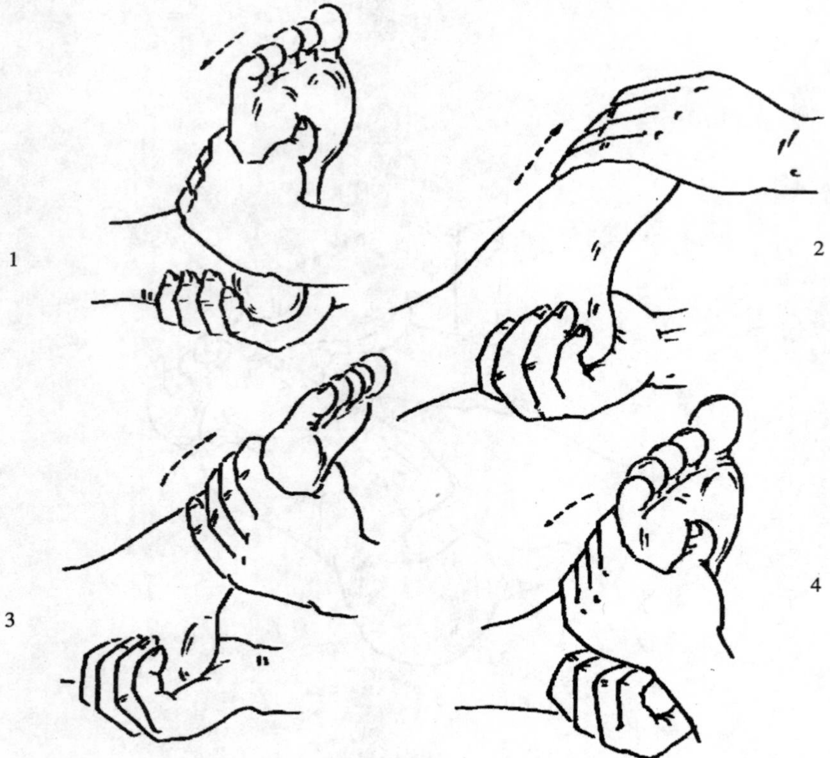

Extension and flexion technique of the ankle.

Manipulation

Grip the dorsum of foot with four finger-pulps and press Yongquan (KI 1) with the thumb. Then place the thumb and index finger of the other hand on Shuiquan (KI 5) located below mdeial malleolus and Pucan (BL 61) located below lateral malleolus. Rotate the foot clockwise and counterclockwise as well as bend the foot back and forth by the hand, meanwhile press and knead the acupoints involved. Repeat the manipulation for 3-5 minutes.

Points

1. Yongquan (KI 1): On the sole, in the depression when the foot is in plantar flexion, approximately at the junction of the anterior one third and posterior two thirds of the sole.

2. Shuiquan (KI 5): 1 *cun* directly below the depression between the tip of the medial malleolus and tendo calcaneus.

3. Pucan (BL 61): Directly below the depression between the external malleolus and tendo calcaneus, at the junction of red and white skin.

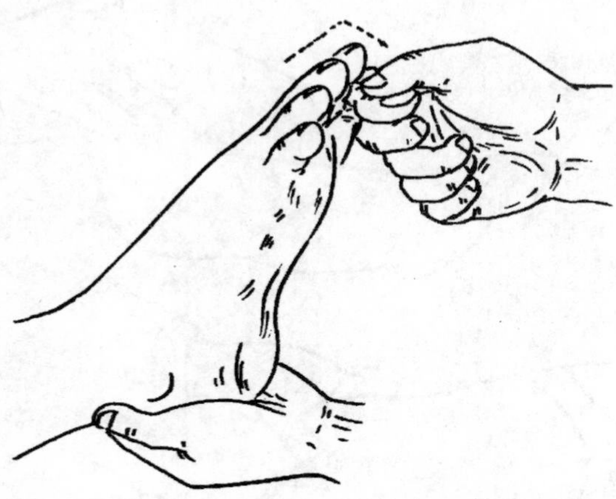

Rotation technique of the big toe.

Manipulation

Use one hand to hold the ankle with the thumb pressing Kunlun (BL 60) and the four fingers pressing Taixi (KI 3). At the same time, pull, bend down and rotate the big toe with the thumb and index finger of the other hand. Repeat the manipulation for 2-5 minutes.

Points

1. Kunlun (BL 60): In the depression between the external malleolus and tendo calcaneus.

2. Taixi (KI 3): In the depression between the medial malleolus and tendo calcaneus.

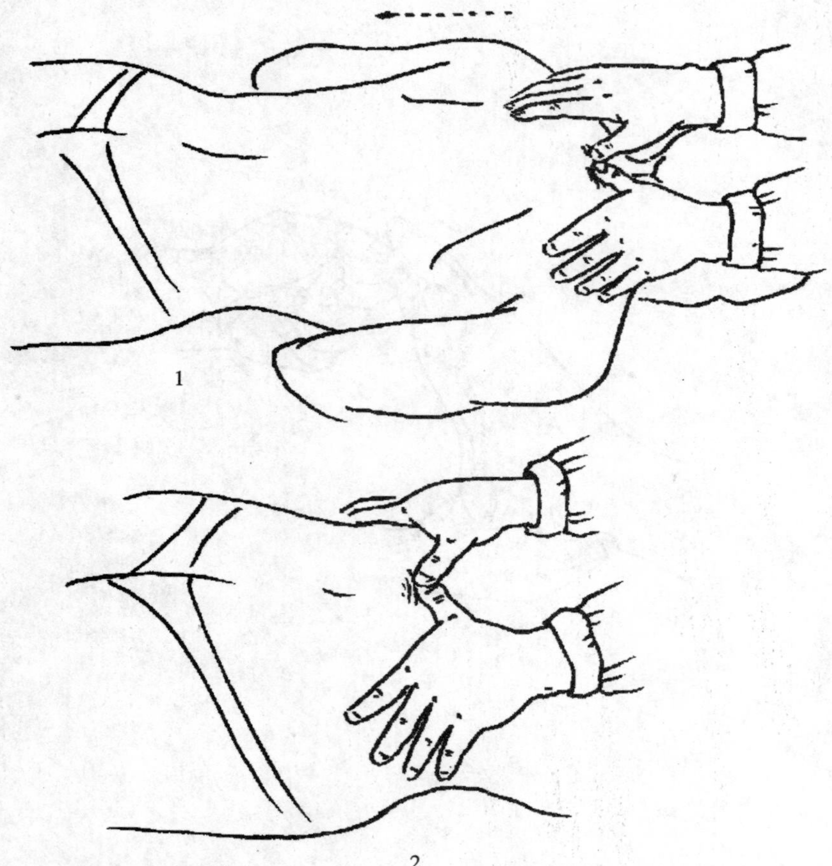

1

2

Pushing technique on Dazhui (GV 14) and Yangguan (GV 3).

Manipulation

Place two thumbs on Dazhui (GV 14), knead the point for 1-2 minutes, then push down along the spine (Governor Vessel) to Yaoyangguan (GV 3), knead the point for 1-2 minutes. Repeat the manipulation for 2-3 times.

Points

1. Dazhui (GV 14): Below the spinous process of the seventh cervical vertebra.

2. Yaoyangguan (GV 3): Below the spinous process of the fourth lumbar vertebra.

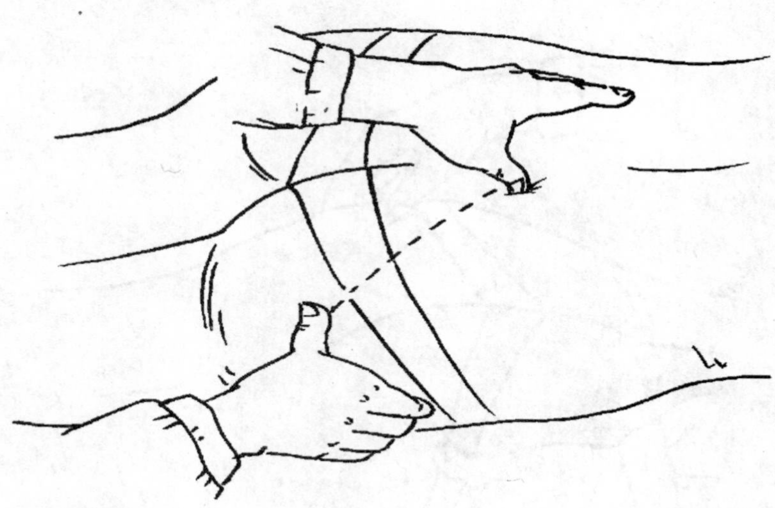

Pushing technique on the buttock.

Manipulation

Place a thumb on Xiaochangshu (BL 27), press and push diagonally downwards past Baohuang (BL 53) and stop at Huantiao (GB 30). Repeat the manipulation with two thumbs massaging alternately for 3-5 minutes.

Points

1. Xiaochangshu (BL 27): At the level of the first posterior sacral foramen and 1.5 *cun* lateral to the posterior midline.

2. Baohuang (BL 53): At the level of the second posterior sacral foramen and 3 *cun* lateral to the posterior midline.

3. Huantiao (GB 30): At the junction of the lateral 1/3 and medial 2/3 of the distance between the great trochanter and the hiatus of the sacrum.

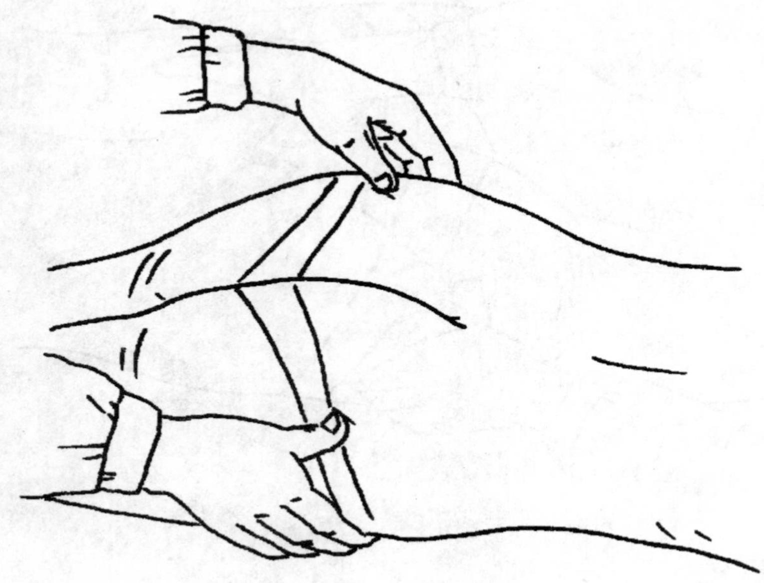

Pressing technique on Huantiao (GB 30).

Manipulation

Lay the two thumbs respectively on Huantiao (GB 30), let other four fingers of both hands grip the sides of the buttocks. Press both points for 1-3 minutes.

Points

Huantiao (GB 30): At the junction of the lateral 1/3 and medial 2/3 of the distance between the great trochanter and the hiatus of the sacrum.

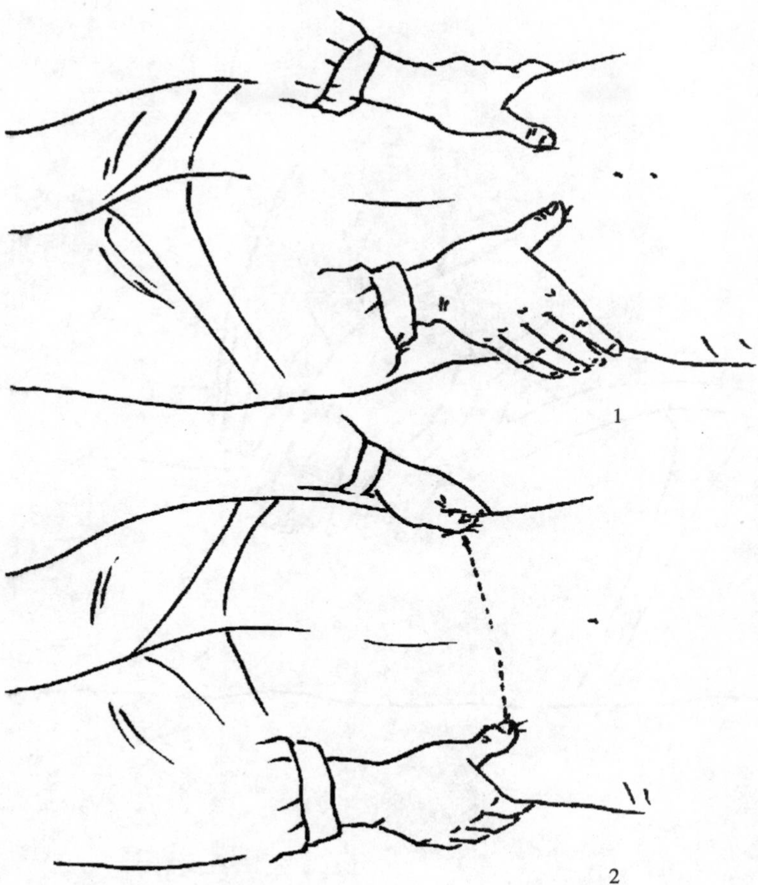

Lateral thumb pushing technique on the lumbar region.

Manipulation

Place two thumbs respectively on bilateral Shenshu (BL 23), and grip around the waist with other four fingers. Conduct pushing technique starting at Shenshu (BL 23), moving laterally from the middle of the back to the side of the back, and stop at Daimai (GB 26). Repeat the manipulation for 1-3 minutes.

Points

1. Shenshu (BL 23): At the level of the lower border of the spinous process of the second lumbar vertebra and 1.5 *cun* lateral to the posterior midline.

2. Daimai (GB 26): Directly below the free end of the eleventh rib, at the level with the umbilicus.

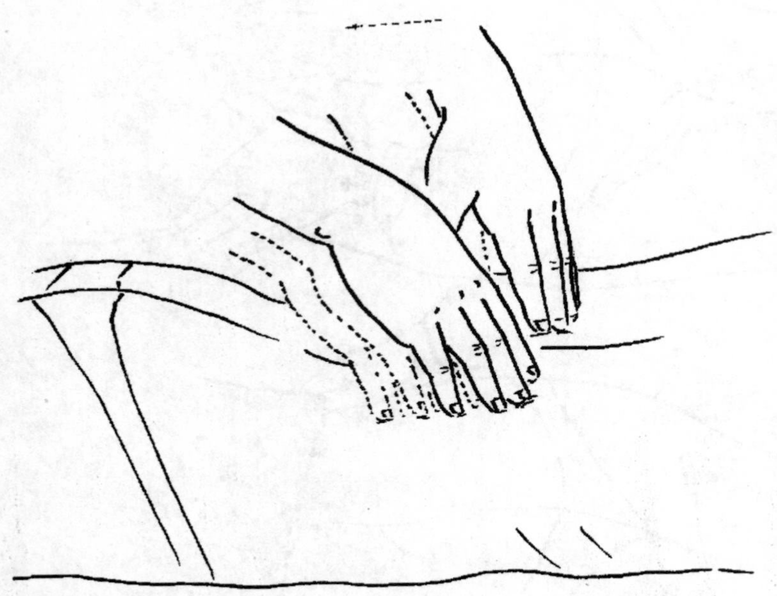

Straight pushing technique on the lumbar region for reinforcing *qi*.

Manipulation

Place four fingers on Shenshu (BL 23), Qihaishu (BL 24) and Dachangshu (BL 25). Then push and knead each acupoint for 1-3 minutes.

Points

1. Shenshu (BL 23): At the level of the lower border of the spinous process of the second lumbar vertebra and 1.5 *cun* lateral to the posterior midline.

2. Qihaishu (BL 24): At the level of the lower border of the spinous process of the third lumbar vertebra and 1.5 *cun* lateral to the posterior midline.

3. Dachangshu (BL 25): At the level of the lower border of the spinous process of the fourth lumbar vertebra and 1.5 *cun* lateral to the posterior midline.

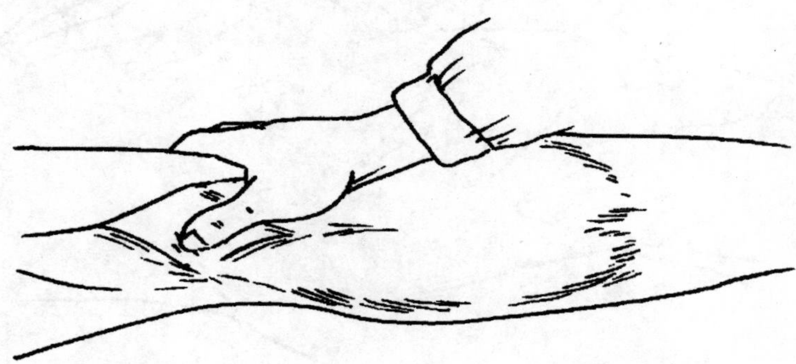

Stationary circular pressing technique on Weizhong (BL 40).

Manipulation

Place a thumb on Weizhong (BL 40) and vigorously press and knead the point for 3-5 minutes.

Points

Weizhong (BL 40): Midpoint of the transverse crease of the popliteal fossa.

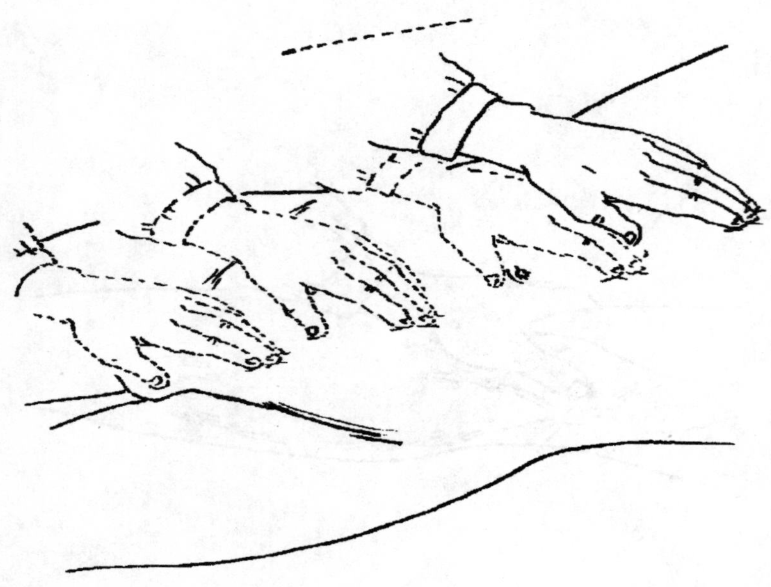

Pressing technique along the midline of the abdomen.

Manipulation

Place four fingertips on Shangwan (CV 13). Press along the midline of the abdomen (Conception Vessel) past Xiawan (CV 10), Guanyuan (CV 4) and stop at Qugu (CV 2). Repeat the manipulation for 1-3 minutes.

Points

1. Shangwan (CV 13): On the midline of the abdomen, 5 *cun* above the umbilicus.

2. Xiawan (CV 10): On the midline of the abdomen, 2 *cun* above the umbilicus.

3. Guanyuan (CV 4): On the midline of the abdomen, 3 *cun* below the umbilicus.

4. Qugu (CV 2): On the midline of the abdomen, 5 *cun* below the umbilicus.

Triceps Muscle and Achilles' Tendon Sprain

Clinical Manifestations

The patient is crippled with local swelling, distention, pain and tenderness; the pain is aggravated by walking, running and jumping with functional disturbance of plantar-flexion.

Differentiation of syndromes:

A. Severe muscle sprain type: Distending pain of the affected side, motor impairment due to severe pain, the pain becoming worse particularly when extending the knee joint, weakness and flaccidity of the foot.

B. Severe Achilles' tendon sprain type: Local swelling and pain extending to the dorsum of the foot, especially when the heel touching the ground, motor impairment of the ankle, severe pain upon dorsiflexion.

Treatment Principle

Removing the obstruction from the meridians, relieving the spasm and pain.

Tuina Techniques

A. Stationary circular pressing technique on Weizhong (BL 40).

B. Stationary circular pressing technique on Chengshan (BL 57).

C. Pressing technique along the lower leg.

D. Pressing technique on Achilles' tendon.

E. Holding technique on Kunlun (BL 60).

F. Extension and flexion techniques of the ankle.

(Tuina treatment is forbidden within 2 days of injury, during which period cold external application should be adopted 2-3 times a day at the local region.)

Addition or Subtraction Techniques

A. Severe muscle sprain type:

Addition: 1. Kneading and pinching techniques along the medial aspect of the lower leg. 2. Stationary circular pressing technique on Zusanli (ST 36).

B. Severe Achilles' tendon sprain type:

Addition: 1. Stationary circular pressing technique on Sanyinjiao (SP 6). 2. Stationary circular pressing technique on Xuanzhong (GB 39).

Subtraction: Extension and flexion techniques of the ankle.

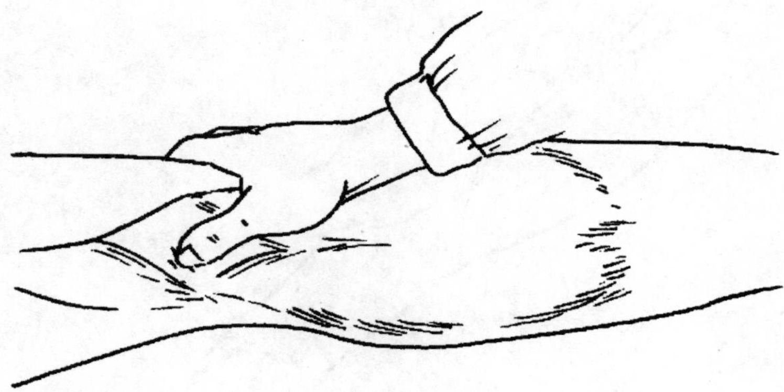

Stationary circular pressing technique on Weizhong (BL 40).

Manipulation

Place a thumb on Weizhong (BL 40) and vigorously press and knead the point for 3-5 minutes.

Points

Weizhong (BL 40): Midpoint of the transverse crease of the popliteal fossa.

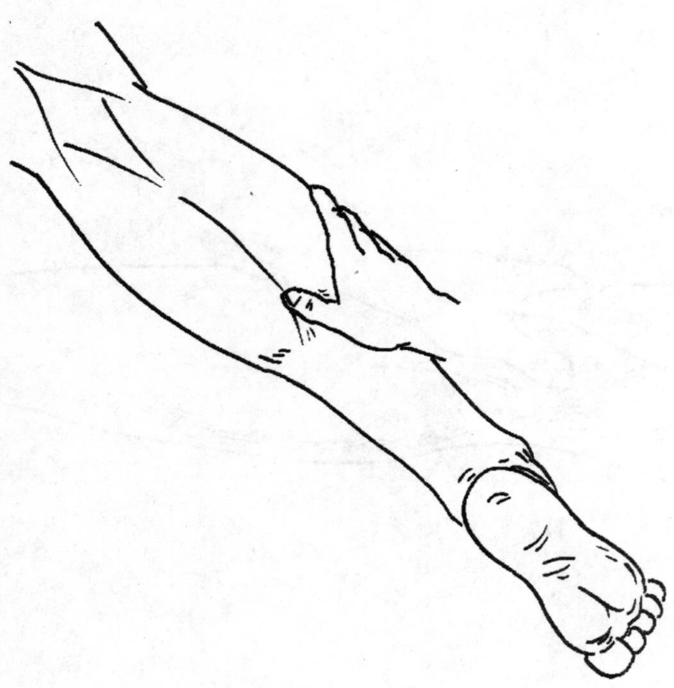

Stationary circular pressing technique on Chengshan (BL 57).

Manipulation

Place a thumb on Chengshan (BL 57) and other fingers on the outside of the shank. Press and knead forcefully for 2-3 minutes.

Points

Chengshan (BL 57): In the top of the depression of the belly of m. gastrocnemius.

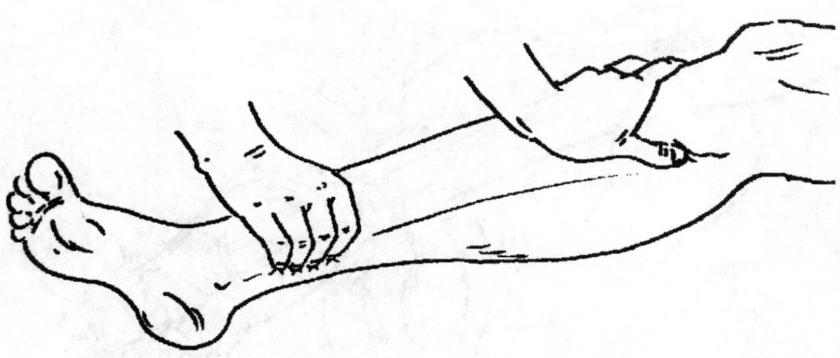

Pressing technique on the lower leg.

Manipulation

Place one thumb on Yinlingquan (SP 9) and the other four fingers on the side of the leg. Place the four fingertips of other hand on Sanyinjiao (SP 6) and lougu (SP 7). Press the points simultaneously 3-5 times, each time should last 15-30 seconds.

Points

1. Yinlingquan (SP 9): On the lower border of the medial condyle of the tibia, in the depression on the medial border of the tibia.

2. Sanyinjiao (SP 6): 3 *cun* directly above the tip of the medial malleolus, on the posterior border of the medial aspect of the tibia.

3. Lougu (SP 7): 3 *cun* directly above Sanyinjiao (SP 6).

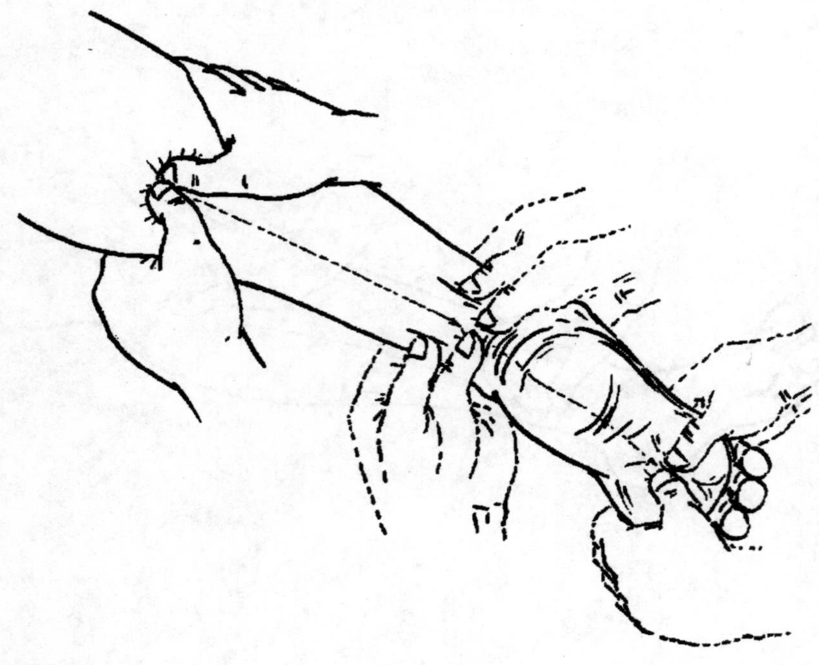

Pressing technique on Achilles' tendon.

Manipulation

Place two thumbs on Chengshan (BL 57), press downwards to the Achilles' tendon. At the tendon press fourcefully for 10-30 seconds. Then continue pressing along the bottom of the foot until Yongquan (KI 1) is reached. Repeat the manipulation for 3-5 times.

Points

1. Chengshan (BL 57): In the top of the depression of the belly of m. gastrocnemius.

2. Yongquan (KI 1): On the sole, in the depression when the foot is in plantar flexion, approximately at the junction of the anterior one third and posterior two thirds of the sole.

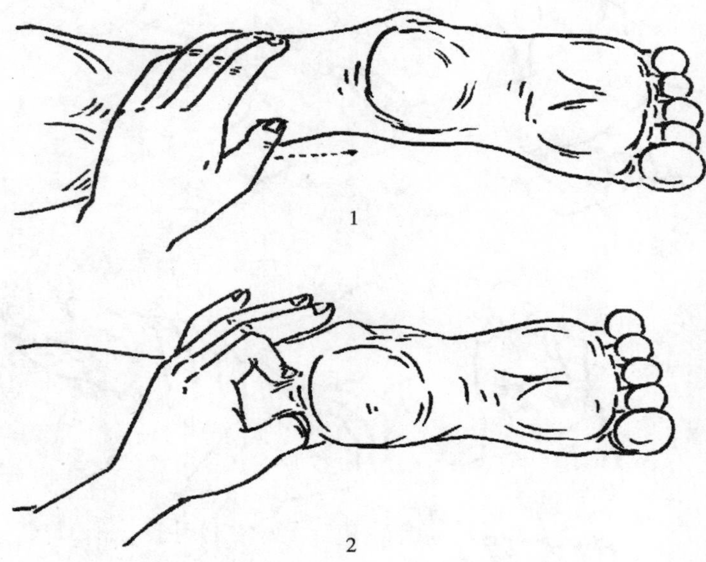

Holding technique on Kunlun (BL 60).

Manipulation

Place the thumb tip and index finger tip respectively on Sanyinjiao (SP 6) and Xuanzhong (GB 39), press down to Taixi (KI 3) and Kunlun (BL 60). Then hold firmly and lift the Achilles' tendon for 3-5 times.

Points

1. Sanyinjiao (SP 6): 3 *cun* directly above the tip of the medial malleolus, on the posterior border of the medial aspect of the tibia.

2. Xuanzhong (GB 39): 3 *cun* above the tip of the external malleolus, in the depression between the anterior border of the fibula and the tendons of m. peroneus longus and brevis.

3. Taixi (KI 3): In the depression between the medial malleolus and tendo calcaneus.

4. Kunlun (BL 60): In the depression between the external malleolus and tendo calcaneus.

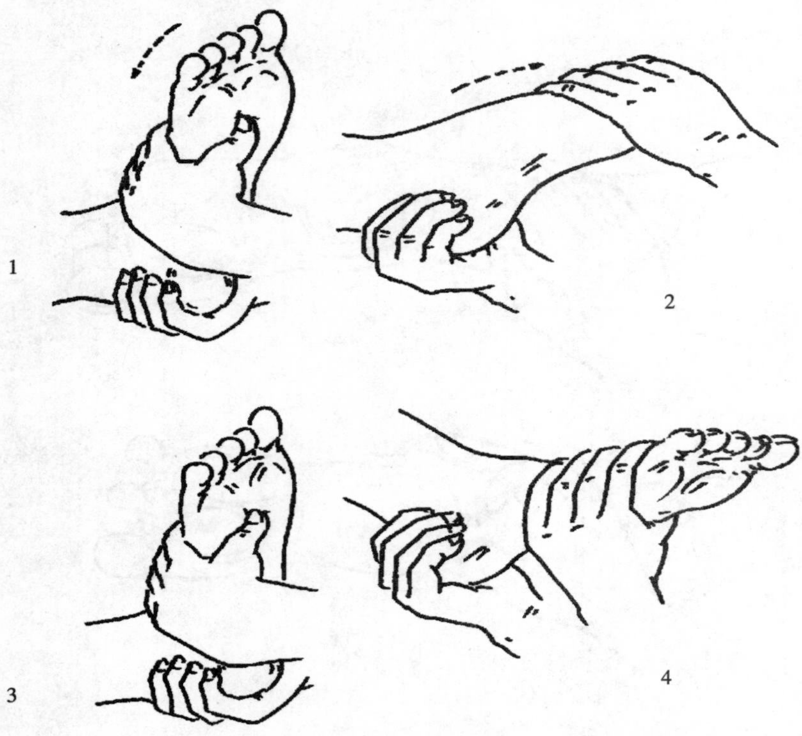

Extension and flexion technique of the ankle.

Manipulation

Grip the dorsum of foot with four finger-pulps and press Yongquan (KI 1) with the thumb. Place the thumb and index finger of the other hand on Shuiquan (KI 5) located below the medial malleolus and Pucan (BL 61) located below the lateral malleolus. Rotate the foot clockwise and counterclockwise as well as bend the foot back and forth by the hand, meanwhile press and knead the acupoints involved. Repeat the manipulation for 3-5 minutes.

Points

1. Yongquan (KI 1): On the sole, in the depression when the foot is in plantar flexion, approximately at the junction of the anterior one third and posterior two thirds of the sole.

2. Shuiquan (KI 5): 1 *cun* directly below the depression between the tip of the medial malleolus and tendo calcaneus.

3. Pucan (BL 61): Directly below the depression between the external malleolus and tendo calcaneus, at the junction of red and white skin.

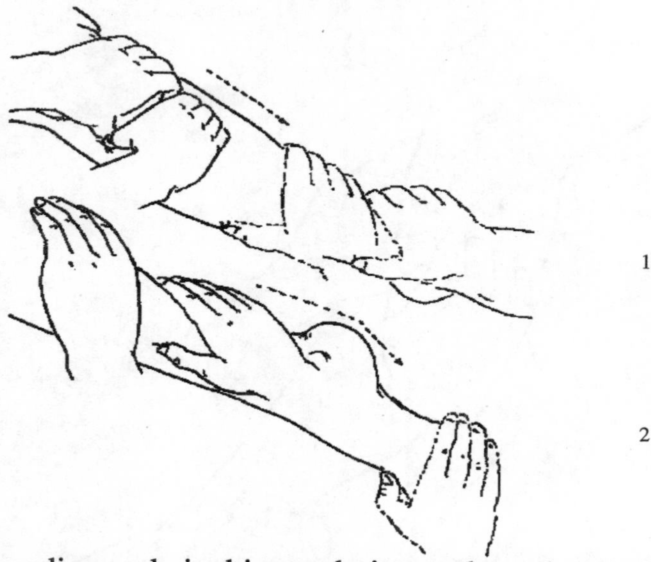

Kneading and pinching techniques along the medial aspect of the lower leg.

Manipulation

Place four fingers of both hands on Yinlingquan (SP 9) and Diji (SP 8) and two thumbs on Yanglingquan (GB 34), press and knead these points. Then use one hand to knead and pinch along the medial aspect of the shank past Sanyinjiao (SP 6) and stop at Shangqiu (SP 5). Repeat the manipulation for 3-5 times. Then from Shangqiu (SP 5) rub downwards past Gongsun (SP 4), stop at Yinbai (SP 1) and press the big toe. Repeat the massage for 5-10 times.

Points

1. Yinlingquan (SP 9): On the lower border of the medial condyle of the tibia, in the depression on the medial border of the tibia.
2. Diji (SP 8): 3 *cun* directly below Yinlingquan (SP 9).
3. Yanglingquan (GB 34): In the depression anterior and inferior to the head of the fibula.
4. Sanyinjiao (SP 6): 3 *cun* directly above the tip of the medial malleolus, on the posterior border of the medial aspect of the tibia.
5. Shangqiu (SP 5): In the depression distal and inferior to the medial malleolus.
6. Gongsun (SP 4): In the depression distal and inferior to the base of the first metatarsal bone.
7. Yinbai (SP 1): On the medial side of the great toe, 0.1 *cun* posterior to the corner of the nail.

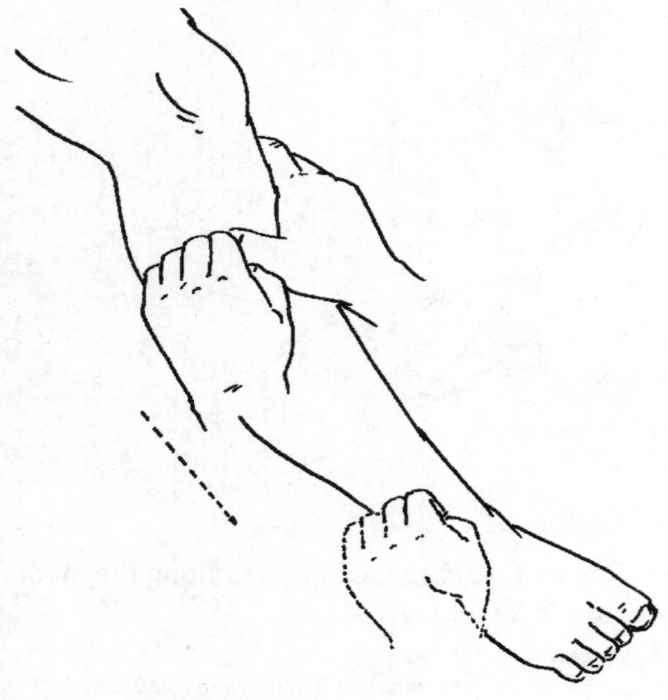

Stationary circular pressing technique on Zusanli (ST 36).

Manipulation

Place a thumb on Zusanli (ST 36), then press and knead the point. At the same time, flex four fingers of the other hand and place them on Yanglingquan (GB 34), and push downwards to Xuanzhong (GB 39). Repeat the manipulation for 1-2 minutes.

Points

1. Zusanli (ST 36): One finger-breadth lateral to the anterior crest of the tibia, in m. tibialis anterior.

2. Yanglingquan (GB 34): In the depression anterior and inferior to the head of the fibula.

3. Xuanzhong (GB 39): 3 *cun* above the tip of the external malleolus, in the depression between the anterior border of the fibula and the tendons of m. peroneus longus and brevis.

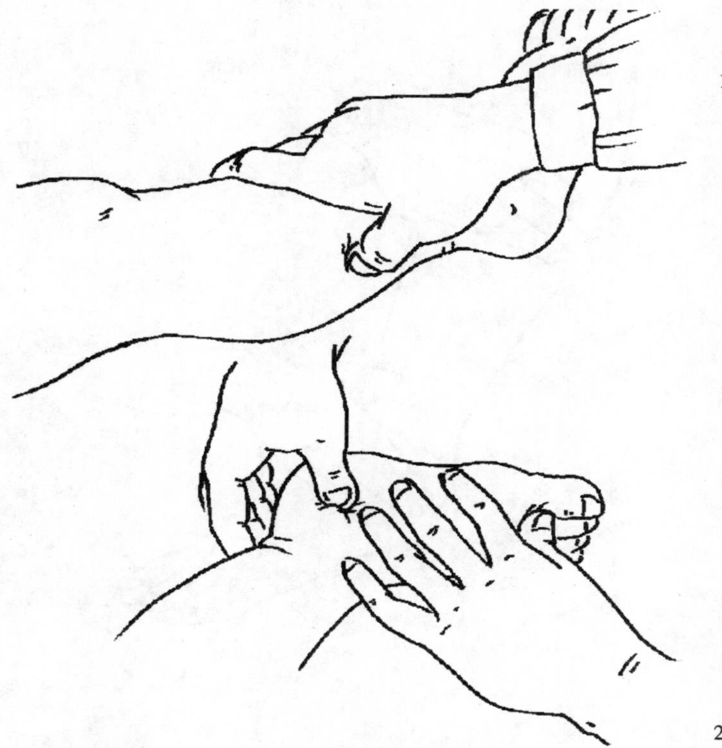

Stationary circular pressing technique on Sanyinjiao (SP 6).

Manipulation

Place a thumb tip on Sanyinjiao (SP 6), press and knead the point for 3-5 minutes. Then move the thumb tip to Zhaohai (KI 6), meanwhile place the other thumb tip on Taichong (LR 3). Press and knead the two points at the same time for 1-3 minutes.

Points

1. Sanyinjiao (SP 6): 3 *cun* directly above the tip of the medial malleolus, on the posterior border of the medial aspect of the tibia.
2. Zhaohai (KI 6): In the depression of the lower border of the medial malleolus.
3. Taichong (LR 3): On the dorsum of the foot, in the depression distal to the junction of the first and second metatarsal bones.

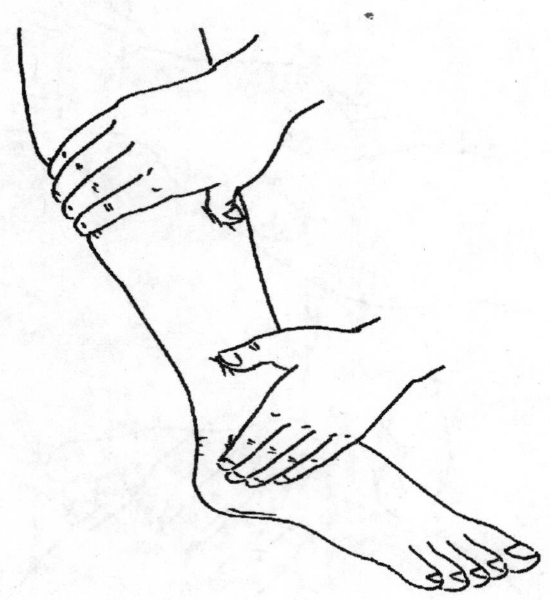

Stationary circular pressing technique on Xuanzhong (GB 39).

Manipulation

Place one thumb on Xuanzhong (GB 39), the other thumb on Tiaokou (ST 38), and the four finger-pulps on Chengshan (BL 57). Press and knead the points simultaneously for 3-5 minutes.

Points

1. Xuanzhong (GB 39): 3 *cun* above the tip of the external malleolus, in the depression between the anterior border of the fibula and the tendons of m. peroneus longus and brevis.

2. Tiaokou (ST 38): 5 *cun* directly below the anterior crest of the tibia and one finger-breadth lateral to the tibia.

3. Chengshan (BL 57): In the top of the depression of the belly of m. gastrocnemius.

Sprain of Ankle

Clinical Manifestations

The sprain, which occurs frequently on the lateral aspect of the ankle and rarely of the medial aspect, happens suddenly with severe pain, redness and swelling of the ankle. The pain is aggravated by walking, moving of the joint or weight lifting.

A. Mild injury type: New injury with slight local swelling and muscle tenderness, redness and purple discolouration of the local skin.

B. Blood stagnation type with swelling and distention: Local region with strong redness and swelling, obvious distending pain, blue and purple skin, difficult flexion and extension of the joint.

Treatment Principle

Activating blood circulation and dispelling the stasis, relieving swelling and pain.

Tuina Techniques

A. Stationary circular pressing technique on Xuanzhong (GB 39).

B. Nipping technique on Jiexi (ST 41).

C. Pushing technique along the lateral aspect of the foot.

D. Combing technique on the dorsum of the foot.

(Within 24 hours of sprain, conduct local external cold application.)

Addition or Subtraction Techniques

A. Mild injury type:

Addition: 1. Pressing technique on Achilles' tendon. 2. Ankle rotation technique.

B. Blood stagnation type with swelling and distention:

Addition: 1. Pressing technique along the lower leg. 2. Extension and flexion technique of the ankle.

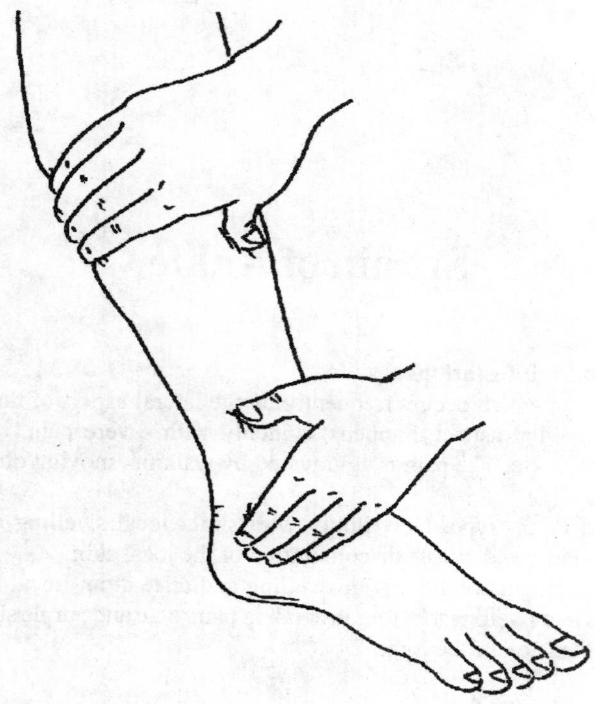

Stationary circular pressing technique on Xuanzhong (GB 39).

Manipulation

Place one thumb on Xuanzhong (GB 39), the other thumb on Tiaokou (ST 38), and the four finger-pulps on Chengshan (BL 57). Press and knead the points simultaneously for 3-5 minutes.

Points

1. Xuanzhong (GB 39): 3 *cun* above the tip of the external malleolus, in the depression between the anterior border of the fibula and the tendons of m. peroneus longus and brevis.

2. Tiaokou (ST 38): 5 *cun* directly below the anterior crest of the tibia and one finger-breadth lateral to the tibia.

3. Chengshan (BL 57): In the top of the depression of the belly of m. gastrocnemius.

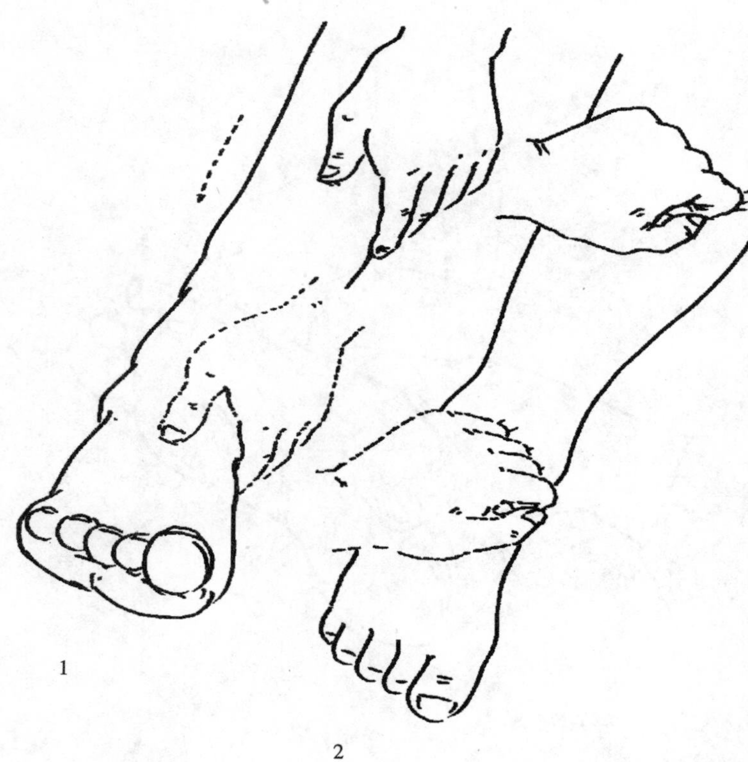

Nipping technique on Jiexi (ST 41).

Manipulation

Place a thumb tip on Fenglong (ST 40) and other four fingers over the outside of the calf. Push downwards from Fenglong (ST 40) to Jiexi (ST 41) and press Jiexi (ST 41) for 30-60 seconds. Repeat the manipulation for 3-5 times. Then place the back of the hollow fist on Fenglong (ST 40), and push down to the dorsum of the foot. Repeat the fist pushing for 5-10 times.

Points

1. Fenglong (ST 40): 5 *cun* directly below the anterior crest of the tibia and two finger-breadth lateral to the tibia.

2. Jiexi (ST 41): On the dorsum of the foot, at the midpoint of the transverse crease of the ankle joint, in the depression between the tendons of m. extensor digitorum longus and hallucis longus.

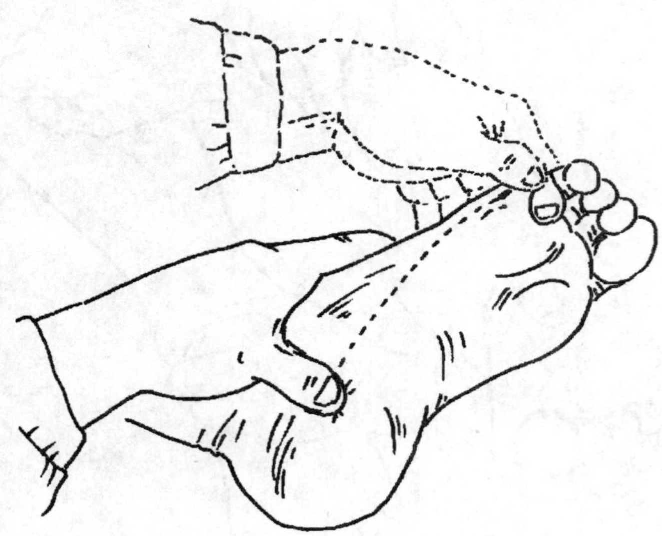

Pushing technique on the lateral aspect of the foot.

Manipulation

Place one thumb on Pucan (BL 61) and the other four fingers on the back of the foot. Push with the thumb along the lateral margin of the foot (Bladder Meridian) to Zhiyin (BL 67), then press the distal section of the little toe to bend it down. Repeat the manipulation 2-5 minutes.

Points

1. Pucan (BL 61):Directly below the depression between the external malleolus and tendo calcaneus, at the junction of red and white skin.

2. Zhiyin (BL 67): On the lateral side of the small toe, about 0.1 *cun* posterior to the corner of the nail.

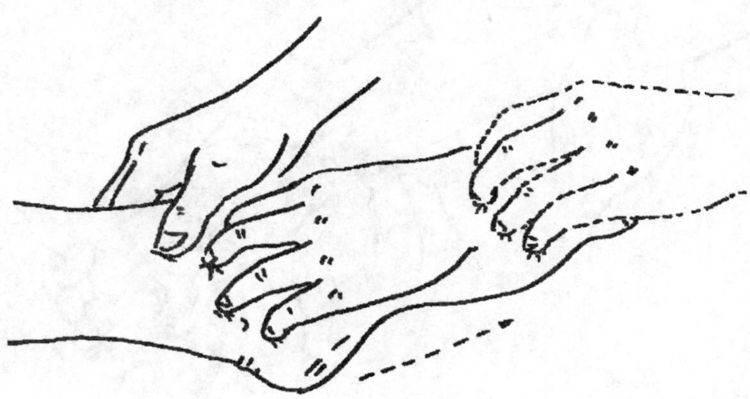

Combing technique on the dorsum of the foot.

Manipulation

Place four finger tips on Jiexi (ST 41) region and comb down to toes. At the same time, press and knead Jiexi (ST 41) by the other thumb. Repeat the manipulation for 1 minute.

Points

Jiexi (ST 41): On the dorsum of the foot, at the midpoint of the transverse crease of the ankle joint, in the depression between the tendons of m. extensor digitorum longus and halluces longus.

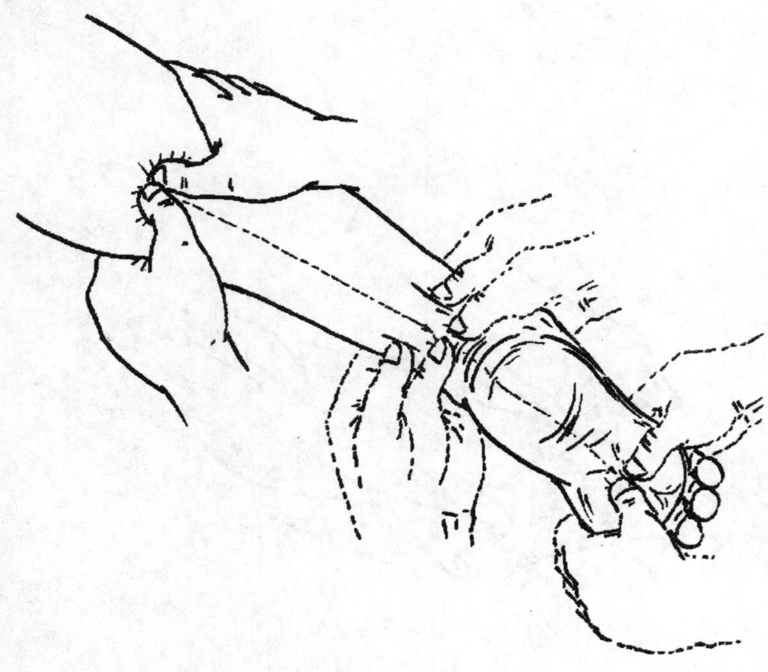

Pressing technique on Achilles' tendon.

Manipulation

Place two thumbs on Chengshan (BL 57), press downwards to the Achilles' tendon. Press the tendon forcefully for 10-30 seconds. Then continue pressing along the bottom of the foot until Yongquan (KI 1) is reached. Repeat the manipulation for 3-5 times.

Points

1. Chengshan (BL 57): In the top of the depression of the belly of m. gastrocnemius.

2. Yongquan (KI 1): On the sole, in the depression when the foot is in plantar flexion, approximately at the junction of the anterior one third and posterior two thirds of the sole.

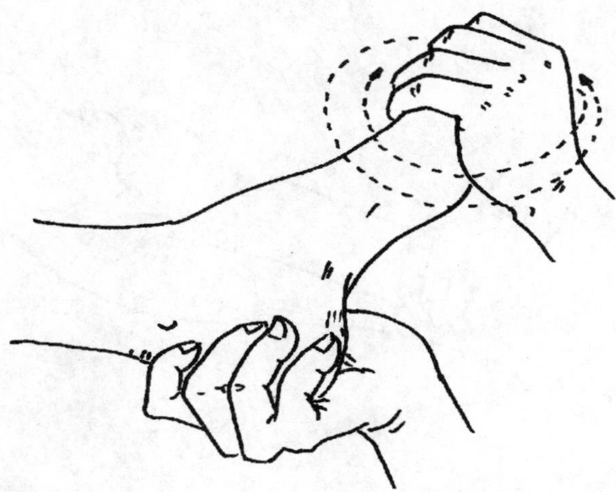

Ankle Rotation technique.

Manipulation

Use one hand to hold the heel region with the thumb and index finger on Pucan (BL 61) and Shuiquan (KI 5). Grab the toes with the other hand and rotate the ankle clockwise and counterclockwise, meanwhile press and knead the points invloved. Repeat the rotation 10-30 times in each direction.

Points

1. Pucan (BL 61): Directly below the depression between the external malleolus and tendo calcaneus, at the junction of red and white skin.

2. Shuiquan (KI 5): 1 *cun* directly below the depression between the tip of the medial malleolus and tendo calcaneus.

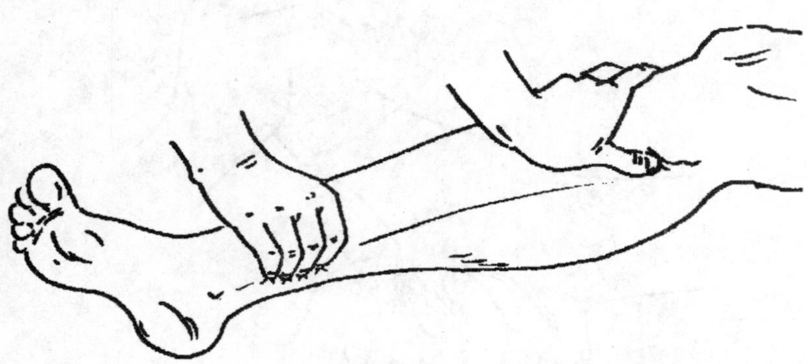

Pressing technique on the lower leg.

Manipulation

Place one thumb on Yinlingquan (SP 9) and the other four fingers on the side of the leg. Place the four fingertips of other hand on Sanyinjiao (SP 6) and lougu (SP 7). Press the points simultaneously 3-5 times, each time should last 15-30 seconds.

Points

1. Yinlingquan (SP 9): On the lower border of the medial condyle of the tibia, in the depression on the medial border of the tibia.

2. Sanyinjiao (SP 6): 3 *cun* directly above the tip of the medial malleolus, on the posterior border of the medial aspect of the tibia.

3. Lougu (SP 7): 3 *cun* directly above Sanyinjiao (SP 6).

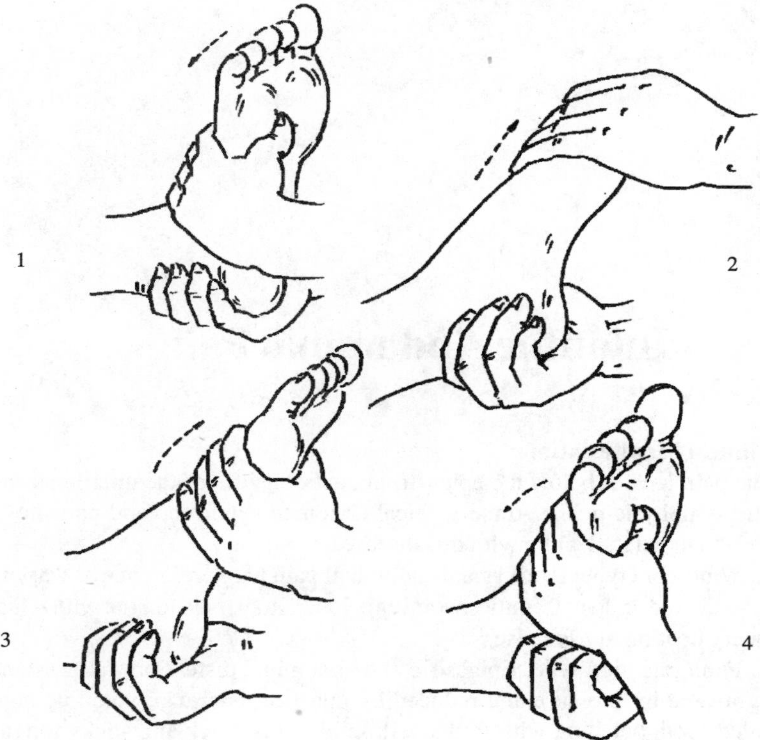

Extension and flexion technique of the ankle.

Manipulation

Grip the dorsum of foot with four finger-pulps and press Yongquan (KI 1) with the thumb. Then place the thumb and index finger of the other hand on Shuiquan (KI 5) located below the medial malleolus and Pucan (BL 61) located below the lateral malleolus. Rotate the foot clockwise and counterclockwise as well as bend the foot back and forth by the hand, meanwhile press and knead the acupoints involved. Repeat the manipulation for 3-5 minutes.

Points

1. Yongquan (KI 1): On the sole, in the depression when the foot is in plantar flexion, approximately at the junction of the anterior one third and posterior two thirds of the sole.

2. Shuiquan (KI 5): 1 *cun* directly below the depression between the tip of the medial malleolus and tendo calcaneus.

3. Pucan (BL 61):Directly below the depression between the external malleolus and tendo calcaneus, at the junction of red and white skin.

Infantile Abdominal Pain

Clinical Manifestations

The pain locates below the epigastrium, at both sides of the umbilicus and above the symphysis pubis. Acute surgical abdomen syndrome and parasitosis should be excluded in dealing with this disease.

A. Wind-cold type: Paroxysmal abdominal pain with preference of warmth and dislike of cold, cold extremities, vomiting, loose stool, pale tongue with white and slippery coating, tense pulse.

B. Food retention type: Epigastric and abdominal distention, fullness and pain aggravated by pressure and reduced by diarrhea, anorexia, vomiting sour and spoiled food, belching with foul smell, fetid flatus, thick and sticky tongue coating, rolling pulse.

Treatment Principle

Dispelling wind and eliminating cold, regulating *qi* and relieving pain.

Tuina Techniques

A. Circular kneading technique on periumbilical region.

B. Stationary circular pressing technique on Zusanli (ST 36).

C. Stationary circular pressing technique on Mingmen (GV 4).

Addition or Subtraction Techniques

A. Wind-cold type:

Addition: 1. Transverse rubbing technique across the umbilicus. 2. Pressing technique on Tianshu (ST 25).

B. Food retention type:

Addition: 1. Diagonal rubbing technique on the hypochondrium. 2. Pressing technique along the medial border of the iliac bone.

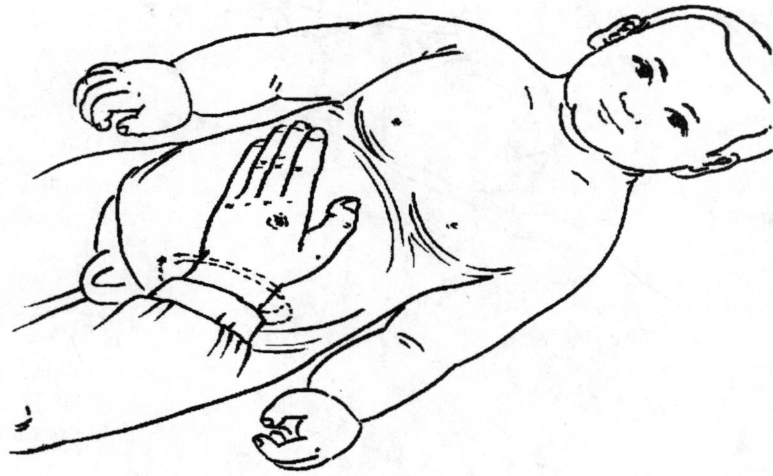

Circular kneading technique on periumbilical region.

Manipulation

Lay the center of a palm on Shenque (CV 8), knead the point clockwise and counterclockwise in each direction, the massage should last 2-3 minutes.

Points

Shenque (CV 8): In the center of the umbilicus.

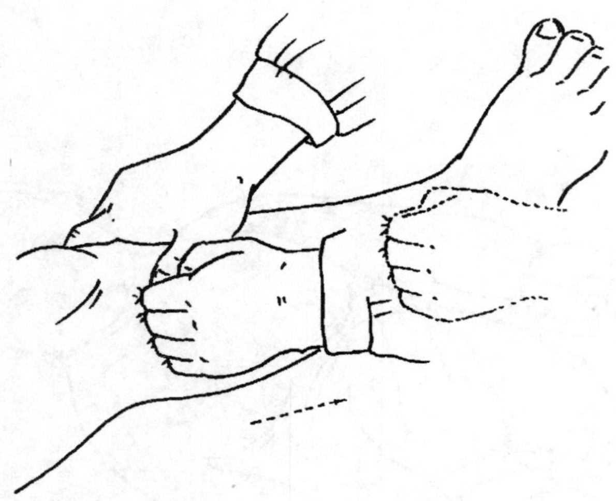

Stationary circular pressing technique on Zusanli (ST 36).

Manipulation

Place a thumb on Zusanli (ST 36), press and knead the point. At the same time, flex four fingers of the other hand and place them on Yanglingquan (GB 34) and push downwards to Xuanzhong (GB 39). Repeat the manipulation for 1-2 minutes.

Points

1. Zusanli (ST 36): One finger-breadth lateral to the anterior crest of the tibia, in m. tibialis anterior.

2. Yanglingquan (GB 34): In the depression anterior and inferior to the head of the fibula.

3. Xuanzhong (GB 39): 3 *cun* above the tip of the external malleolus, in the depression between the posterior border of the fibula and the tendons of m. peroneus longus and brevis.

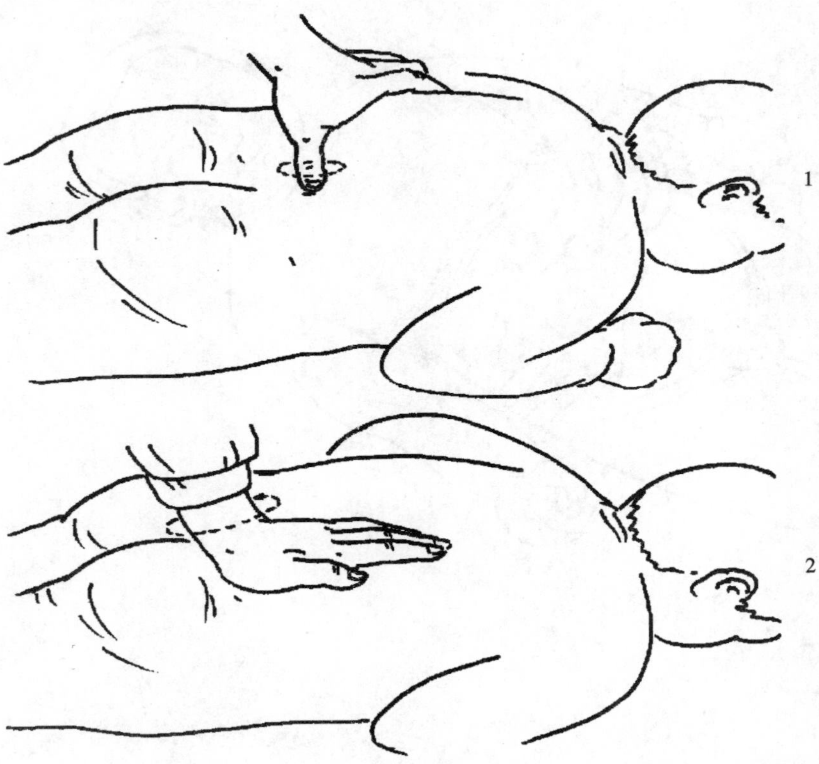

Stationary circular pressing technique on Mingmen (GV 4).

Manipulation

Place a thumb on Mingmen (GV 4), press and knead the point for 2-3 minutes, then place the palm flat on the same area and conduct circular pressing for 1-2 minutes.

Points

Mingmen (GV 4): Below the spinous process of the second lumbar vertebra.

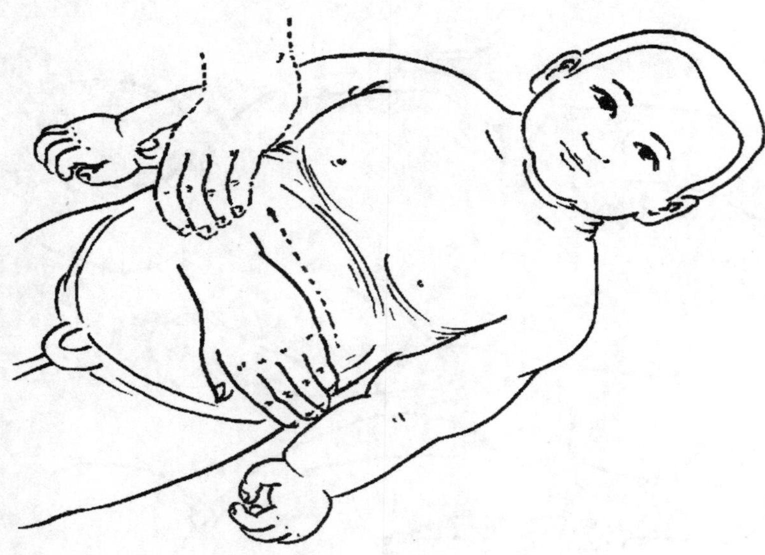

Transverse rubbing technique across the umbilicus.

Manipulation

Place four finger-pulps on one side of Daheng (SP 15) and Fujie (SP 14), rub transversely across the abdomen and past Tianshu (ST 25) and Wailing (ST 26), and stop at Daheng (SP 15) and Fujie (SP 14) on the opposite side. Repeat the manipulation for 2-3 minutes.

Points

1. Daheng (SP 15): 4 *cun* lateral to the center of the umbilicus.
2. Fujie (SP 14): 1.3 *cun* below the umbilicus and 4 *cun* lateral to the midline.
3. Tianshu (ST 25): 2 *cun* lateral to the center of the umbilicus.
4. Wailing (ST 26): 1 *cun* below the center of the umbilicus and 2 *cun* lateral to the midline.

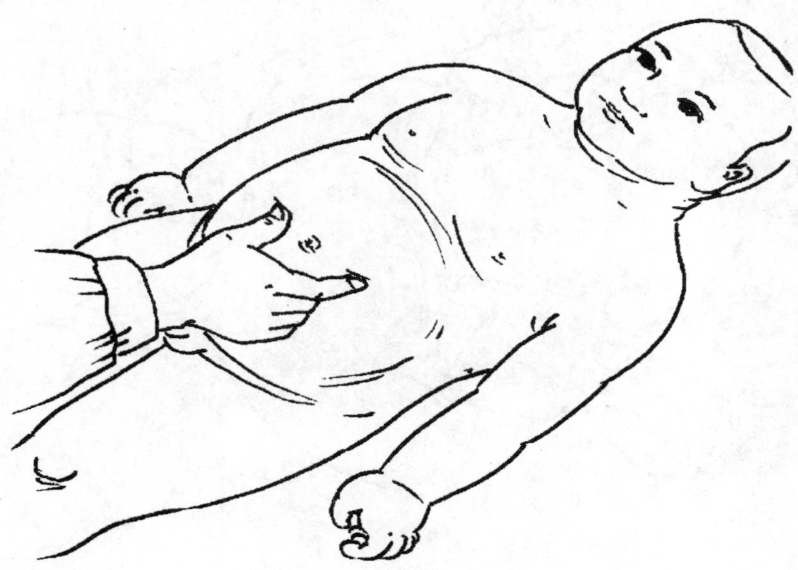

Pressing technique on Tianshu (ST 25).

Manipulation

Place the thumb tip and index finger tip of one hand respectively on bilateral Tianshu (ST 25), press and knead the point forcefully for 3-5 times, each time should last 1-2 minutes.

Points

Tianshu (ST 25): 2 *cun* lateral to the center of the umbilicus.

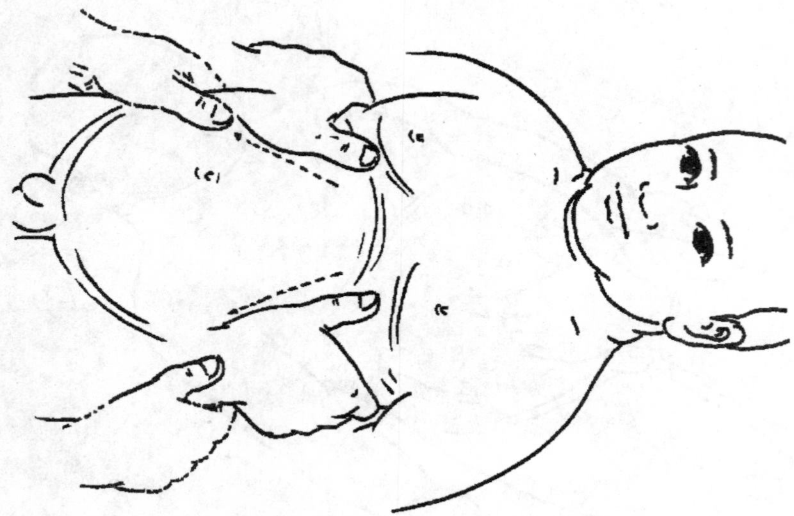

Diagonal rubbing technique on the hypochondrium.

Manipulation

Place two thumbs respectively on bilateral Burong (ST 19) and Chengman (ST 20), rub along the border of rib cage diagonally and stop at both sides of Zhangmen (LR 13). Repeat the manipulation for 3-5 minutes.

Points

1. Burong (ST 19):6 *cun* above the center of the umbilicus and 2 *cun* lateral to the midline.

2. Chengman (ST 20): 5 *cun* above the center of the umbilicus and 2 *cun* lateral to the midline.

3. Zhangmen (LR 13): On the lateral side of the abdomen, below the free end of the eleventh floating rib.

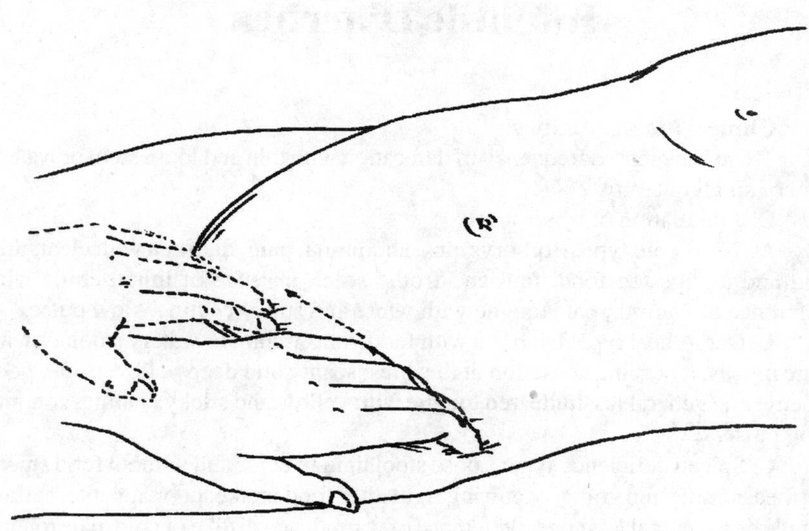

Pressing technique along the medial border of the iliac bone.

Manipulation

Place four fingertips on Wushu (GB 27) on the side of the ilium, and then press and push down to Qichong (ST 30). Repeat the manipulation for 1-2 minutes.

Points

1. Wushu (GB 27): 0.5 *cun* anterior to the anterior superior iliac spine.

2. Qichong (ST 30): 5 *cun* directly below the center of the umbilicus and 2 *cun* lateral to the anterior midline.

Infantile Diarrhea

Clinical Manifestations

There is increased frequency of defecation with thin and loose stool or watery stool of small quantity.

Differentiation of syndromes:

A. Wind-cold type: Borborygmus, abdominal pain, diarrhea with clear, thin fluid and undigested food, foul and frothy stool, absence of thirst, chills with preference of warmth; pale tongue with white and sticky coating, slow pulse.

B. Damp-heat type: Diarrhea with fetid yellow, thin, or watery stool, or with some mucus, a burning sensation at the anus, scanty and deep yellow urine, poor appetite and general lassitude, red tongue with yellow and sticky coating, soft and rapid pulse.

C. Spleen deficiency type: Loose stool light in color and without fetid smell, diarrhea coming and going, occurring right after food intake, poor appetite, sallow complexion, general lassitude, preference of warmth and dislike of cold; pale tongue with white coating, weak pulse.

D. Improper diet type: Distention and fullness in epigastric and abdominal region, diarrhea immediately induced by abdominal pain and relieved after bowel movement; defecation with sour and fetid stool, belching with acid and foul smell; thick and sticky tongue coating, or yellowish coating.

Treatment Principle

Regulating the spleen and stomach, harmonizing the middle energizer to stop diarrhea.

Tuina Techniques

A. Pressing technique along the midline of the abdomen.

B. Pressing technique on Tianshu (ST 25).

C. Circular kneading technique on periumbilical region.

D. Stationary circular pressing technique on Zusanli (ST 36).

E. Pushing technique on the back.

F. Digital pressing technique on the hypochondrium for reinforcing *qi*.

G. Lateral thumb pushing technique on the lumbar region.

H. Stationary circular pressing technique on Changqiang (GV 1).

Addition or Subtraction Techniques

A. Wind-cold type:

Addition: Holding and lifting techniques on the back.

B. Damp-heat type:

Addition: 1. Rubbing and pressing techniques on the hypochondrium. 2. Small relieving *qi* stagnation technique.

Subtraction: 1. Circular kneading technique on periumbilical region. 2. Digital pressing technique on the hypochondrium for reinforcing *qi*.

C. Spleen deficiency type:

Addition: Stationary circular pressing technique on Sanyinjiao (SP 6).

D. Improper diet type:

Addition: 1. Rubbing and pressing techniques on the upper abdomen. 2. Rotation technique of the big toe.

Subtraction: 1. Digital pressing technique on the hypochondrium for reinforcing *qi*.

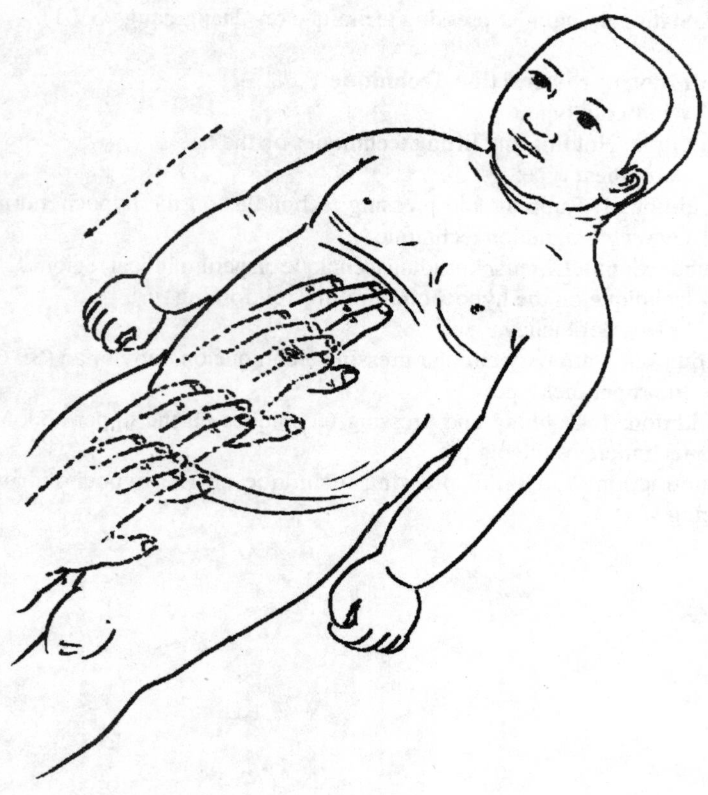

Pressing technique along the midline of the abdomen.

Manipulation

Place four fingertips on Shangwan (CV 13). Slowly press downwards along the midline of the abdomen past Xiawan (CV 10), Guanyuan (CV 4) and stop at Qugu (CV 2). Repeat the manipulation for 1-3 minutes.

Points

1. Shangwan (CV 13): On the midline of the abdomen, 5 *cun* above the umbilicus.

2. Xiawan (CV 10): On the midline of the abdomen, 2 *cun* above the umbilicus.

3. Guanyuan (CV 4): On the midline of the abdomen, 3 *cun* below the umbilicus.

4. Qugu (CV 2): On the midline of the abdomen, 5 *cun* below the umbilicus.

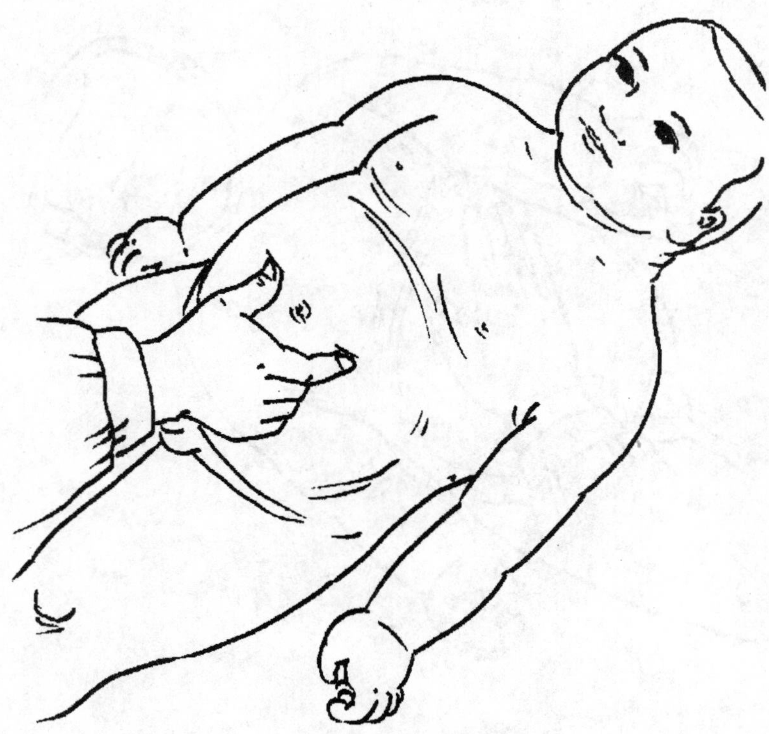

Pressing technique on Tianshu (ST 25).

Manipulation

Place the thumb tip and index finger tip of one hand respectively on bilateral Tianshu (ST 25), press and knead the points forcefully for 3-5 times, each time should last 1-2 minutes.

Points

Tianshu (ST 25): 2 *cun* lateral to the center of the umbilicus.

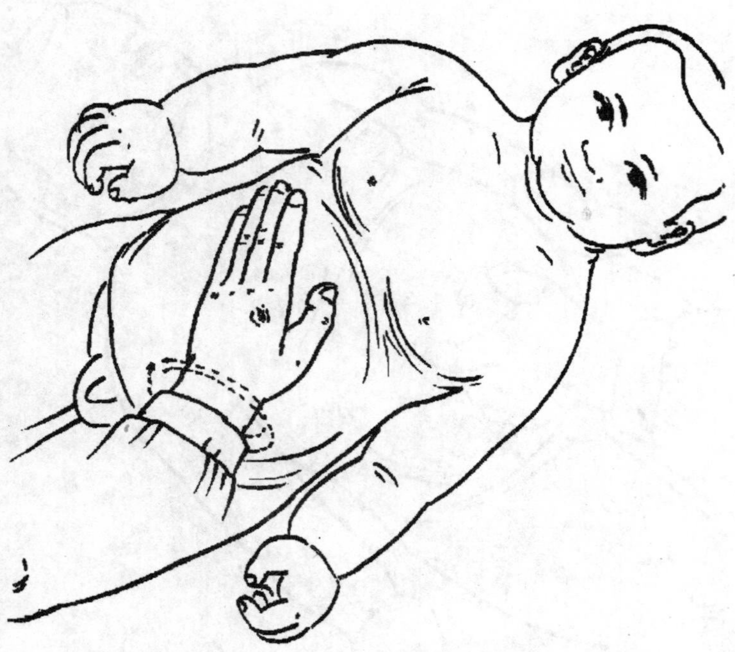

Circular kneading technique on periumbilical region.

Manipulation

Lay the center of a palm on Shenque (CV 8), knead the point clockwise and counterclockwise in each direction, the massage should last 2-3 minutes.

Points

Shenque (CV 8): In the center of the umbilicus.

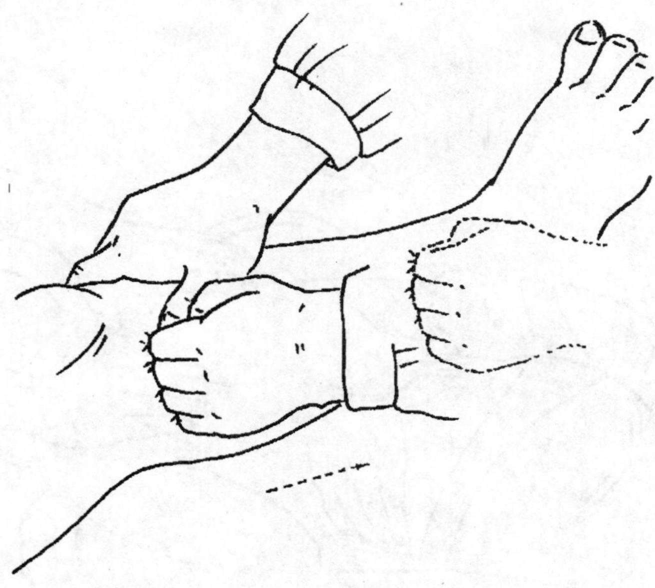

Stationary circular pressing technique on Zusanli (ST 36).

Manipulation

Place a thumb on Zusanli (ST 36), press and knead the point. At the same time, flex four fingers of the other hand and place them on Yanglingquan (GB 34), and push downwards to Xuanzhong (GB 39). Repeat the manipulation for 1-2 minutes.

Points

1. Zusanli (ST 36): One finger-breadth lateral to the anterior crest of the tibia, in m. tibialis anterior.

2. Yanglingquan (GB 34): In the depression anterior and inferior to the head of the fibula.

3. Xuanzhong (GB 39): 3 *cun* above the tip of the external malleolus, in the depression between the posterior border of the fibula and the tendons of m. peroneus longus and brevis.

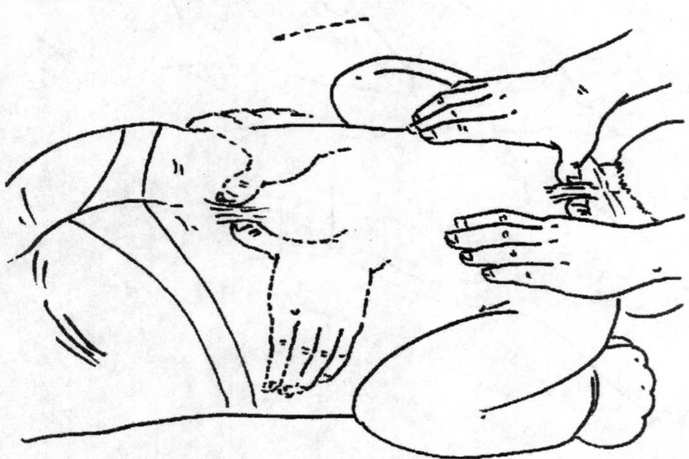

Pushing technique on the back.

Manipulation

Place two thumbs respectively on bilateral Dazhu (BL 11), then squeeze and push straight downwards along both sides of the spine and stop at Dachangshu (BL 25). Repeat the manipulation for 3-5 times.

Points

1. Dazhu (BL 11): At the level of the lower border of the spinous process of the first thoracic vertebra and 1.5 *cun* lateral to the posterior midline.

2. Dachangshu (BL 25): At the level of the lower border of the spinous process of the fourth lumbar vertebra and 1.5 *cun* lateral to the posterior midline.

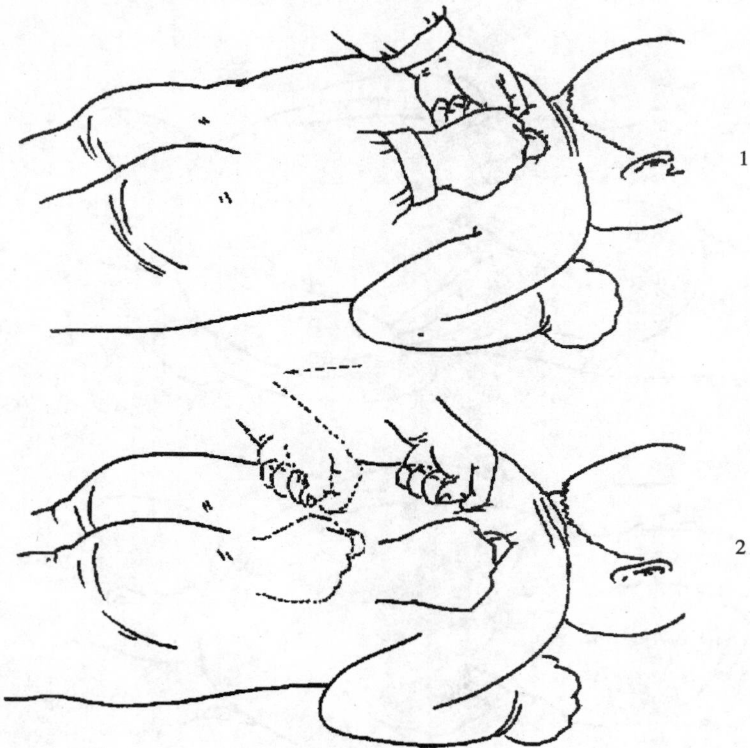

Digital pressing technique on the hypochondrium for reinforcing *qi*.

Manipulation

Place the index finger knuckles of both hands respectively on bilateral Dazhu (BL 11) then press straight downwards along the first line of Bladder Meridian past Xinshu (BL 15) and stop at Geshu (BL 17). Repeat the manipulation for 3-5 times.

Points

1. Dazhu (BL 11): At the level of the lower border of the spinous process of the first thoracic vertebra and 1.5 *cun* lateral to the posterior midline.

2. Xinshu (BL 15): At the level of the lower border of the spinous process of the fifth thoracic vertebra and 1.5 *cun* lateral to the posterior midline.

3. Geshu (BL 17): At the level of the lower border of the spinous process of the seventh thoracic vertebra and 1.5 *cun* lateral to the posterior midline.

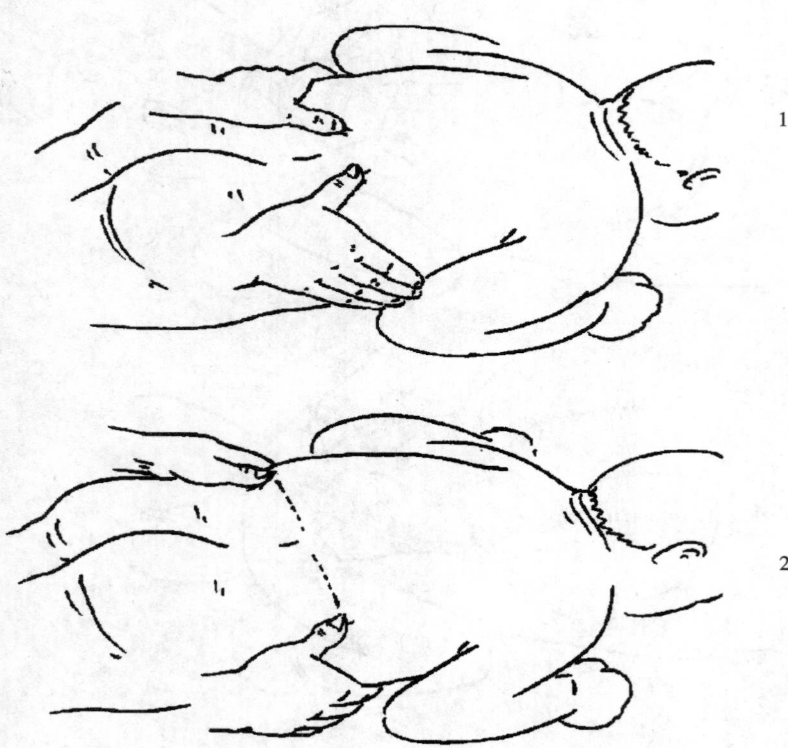

Lateral thumb pushing technique on the lumbar region.

Manipulation

Place two thumbs respectively on bilateral Shenshu (BL 23), and other four fingers around the waist. Then push laterally to the side of the back, and stop at Daimai (GB 26). Repeat the manipulation for 1-3 minutes.

Points

1. Shenshu (BL 23): At the level of the lower border of the spinous process of the second lumbar vertebra and 1.5 *cun* lateral to the posterior midline.

2. Daimai (GB 26): Directly below the free end of the eleventh rib, at the level with the umbilicus.

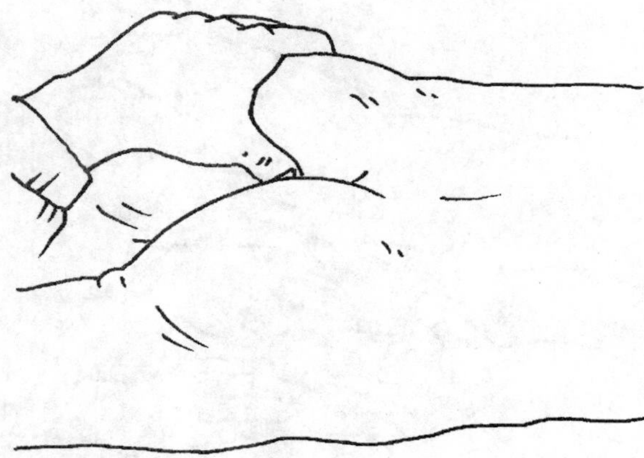

Stationary circular pressing technique on Changqiang (GV 1).

Manipulation

Place the four fingers on the buttock and the thumb on Changqiang (GV 1). Press and knead Changqiang (GV 1) for 1-2 minutes.

Points

Changqiang (GV 1): 0.5 *cun* inferior to the coccyx.

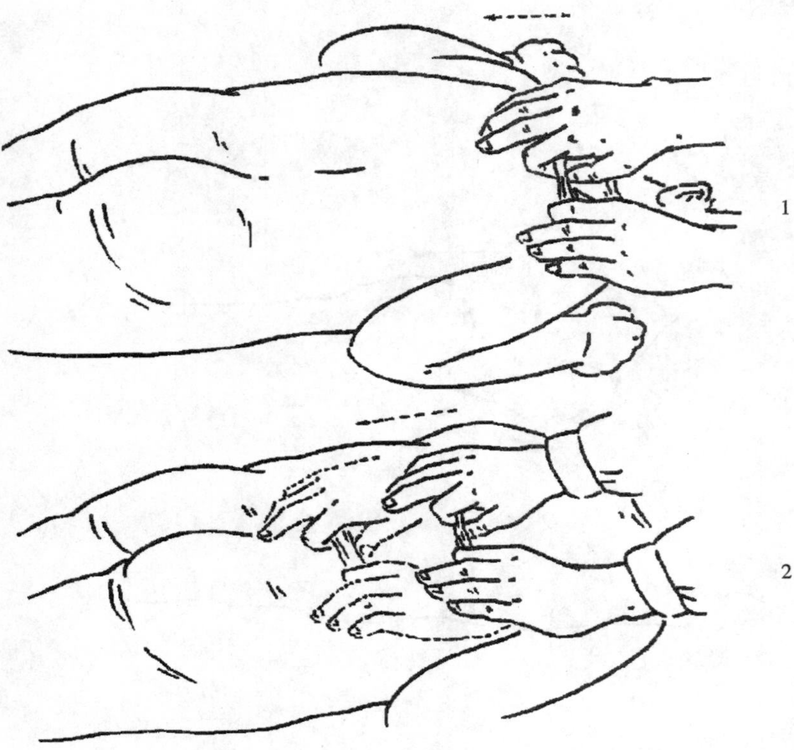

Holding and lifting techniques on the back.

Manipulation

Use the thumbs and index fingers to pinch Dazhu (BL 11) then keep on pinching and pulling up the muscle down the back past Pishu (BL 20) and stop at Guanyuanshu (BL 26). Repeat the manipulation for 3-5 times.

Points

1. Dazhu (BL 11): At the level of the lower border of the spinous process of the first thoracic vertebra and 1.5 *cun* lateral to the posterior midline.

2. Pishu (BL 20): At the level of the lower border of the spinous process of the eleventh thoracic vertebra and 1.5 *cun* lateral to the posterior midline.

3. Guanyuanshu (BL 26):At the level of the lower border of the spinous process of the fifth lumbar vertebra and 1.5 *cun* lateral to the posterior midline.

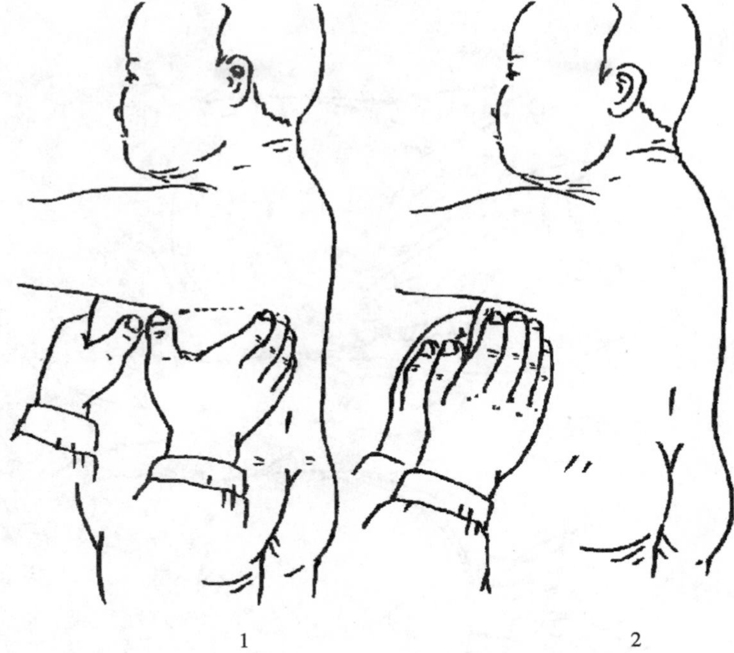

1 2

Rubbing and pressing techniques on the hypochondrium.

Manipulation

Place four finger-pulps of one hand on Burong (ST 19) and Chengman (ST 20) located at the hypochondriac region. Place four finger-pulps of the other hand on Hunmen (BL 47) and Yanggang (BL 48). Press these points for 3-5 seconds. Then rub upward towards the axillary midline where the finger-pulps of both hands finally meet. Repeat the manipulation for 1-3 minutes.

Points

1. Burong (ST 19): 6 *cun* above the umbilicus and 2 *cun* lateral to the midline.
2. Chengman (ST 20): 5 *cun* above the umbilicus and 2 *cun* lateral to the midline.
3. Hunmen (BL 47): At the level of the lower border of the spinous process of the ninth thoracic vertebra, 3 *cun* lateral to the midline.
4. Yanggang (BL 48): At the level of the lower border of the spinous process of the tenth thoracic vertebra, 3 *cun* lateral to the midline.

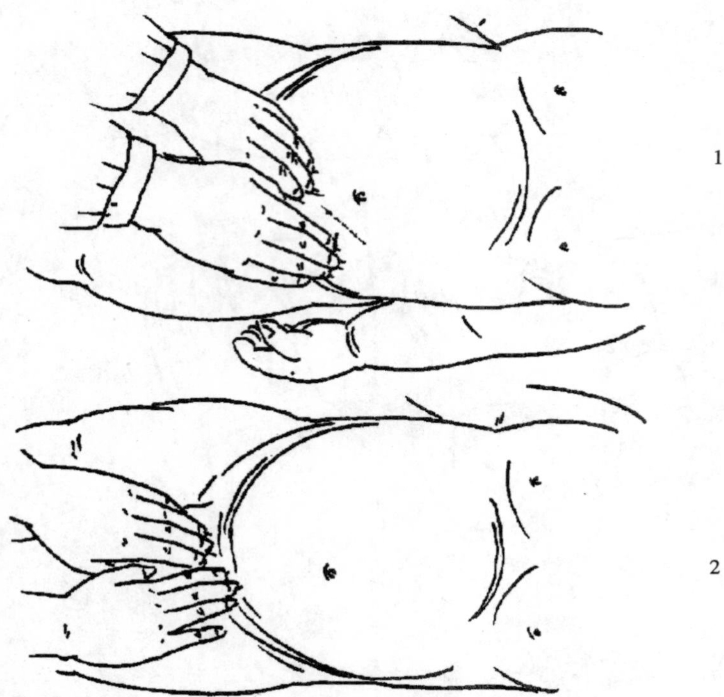

Small relieving *qi* stagnation technique.

Manipulation

Place four finger-pulps of both hands on unilateral Weidao (GB 28) located at the supramedial border of hip bone, then rub and press in an inferior-medial direction down to Qichong (ST 30). Repeat the manipulation for 2-4 minutes.

Points

1. Weidao (GB 28): 1 *cun* anterior and inferior to the anterior superior iliac spine, about 3 *cun* lateral to the anterior midline.

2. Qichong (ST 30): 5 *cun* below and 2 *cun* lateral to the center of the umbilicus.

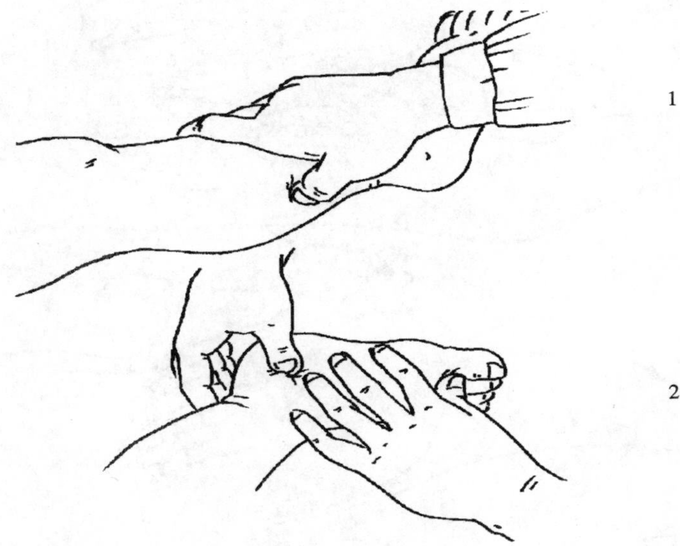

Stationary circular pressing technique on Sanyinjiao (SP 6).

Manipulation

Place a thumb tip on Sanyinjiao (SP 6), press and knead the point for 2-5 minutes. Then move the thumb tip to Zhaohai (KI 6), meanwhile place the other thumb tip on Taichong (LR 3), press and knead the two points at the same time for 1-3 minutes.

Points

1. Sanyinjiao (SP 6): 3 *cun* directly above the tip of the medial malleolus, on the posterior border of the medial aspect of the tibia.
2. Zhaohai (KI 6): In the depression of the lower border of the medial malleolus.
3. Taichong (LR 3): On the dorsum of the foot, in the depression distal to the junction of the first and second metatarsal bones.

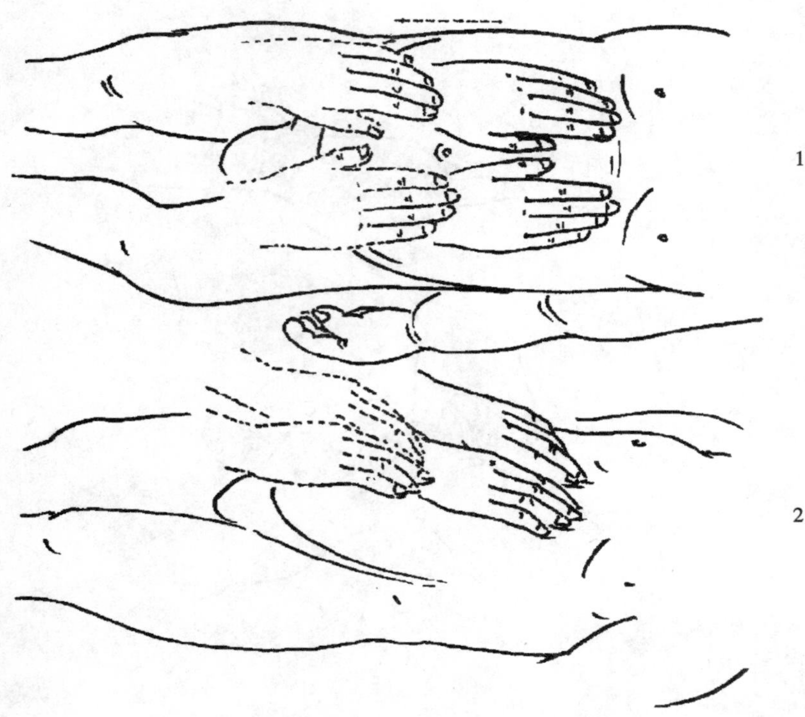

Rubbing and pressing techniques on the upper abdomen.

Manipulation

Place four finger-pulps of both hands on Burong (ST 19) and then rub downwards to Tianshu (ST 25). Repeat the massage for 1-2 minutes, then press Burong (ST 19) and Tianshu (ST 25) for 1-2 minutes.

Points

1. Burong (ST 19): 6 *cun* above the umbilicus and 2 *cun* lateral to the midline.
2. Tianshu (ST 25): 2 *cun* lateral to the center of the umbilicus.

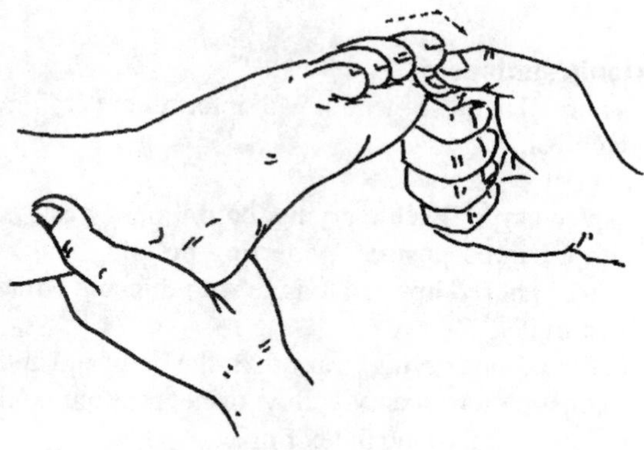

Rotation technique of the big toe.

Manipulation

Use one hand to hold the ankle with the thumb pressing Kunlun (BL 60) and the four fingers pressing Taixi (KI 3). At the same time, pull, bend down and rotate the big toe with the thumb and index finger of the other hand. Repeat the manipulation for 2-5 minutes.

Points

1. Kunlun (BL 60): In the depression between the external malleolus and tendo calcaneus.

2. Taixi (KI 3): In the depression between the medial malleolus and tendo calcaneus.

Infantile Night Crying

Clinical Manifestations

The child is normal at day time, but with intermittent crying at night which often goes until daybreak.

Differentiation of syndromes:

A. Cold in spleen type: Feeble crying, cold limbs, weak suckling, loose stool, sleeping with a curved posture, preferring pressing and kneading at the abdomen, clear urine, light red lips and tongue with thin and white coating, light red vein of the index finger.

B. Heart fire type: Loud crying, warmth of the body and abdomen, flushed face and red lips, constipation, scanty yellow urine, red tongue tip with yellow coating, red and purplish vein of the index finger.

C. Fear and fright type: Sudden onset with continuous nighttime crying, blue and gray complexion, uneasiness, frequent fear and fright, rapid pulse.

Treatment Principle

Warming the spleen and clearing the heart, easing the mind and relieving the crying.

Tuina Techniques

A. Rubbing technique on the back.

B. Holding and lifting techniques on the back.

C. Pushing technique along the Three Yin meridians of Hand on forearm.

D. Opposite pressing technique on Neiguan (PC 6) and Waiguan (TE 5).

E. Stationary circular pressing technique on Laogong (PC 8).

F. Stationary circular pressing technique on Yongquan (KI 1).

Addition or Subtraction Techniques

A. Spleen cold type:

Addition: Squeezing and pushing techniques on the back.

B. Heart fire type:

Addition: Chest extending technique.

2. Squeezing and pushing techniques on the abdomen.

C. Fear and fright type:

Addition: Rubbing and pressing techniques on the upper abdomen.

Subtraction: Pushing technique along the Three Yin meridians of Hand on the forearm.

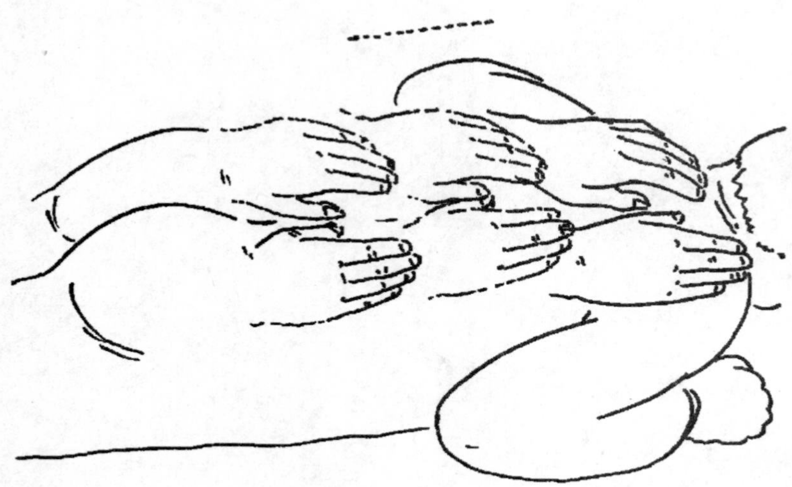

Rubbing technique on the back.

Manipulation

Place both palms on each side of the back, with both thumbs on Dazhui (GV 14), and slowly massage downwards along the spine (Governor Vessel) past Zhiyang (GV 9) and stop at Xuanshu (GV 5), at the same time knead the points of the Governor Vessel along the spine with the thumbs. Repeat the manipulation for 3-5 minutes.

Points

1. Dazhui (GV 14): Below the spinous process of the seventh cervical vertebra.

2. Zhiyang (GV 9): Below the spinous process of the seventh thoracic vertebra.

3. Xuanshu (GV 5): Below the spinous process of the first lumbar vertebra.

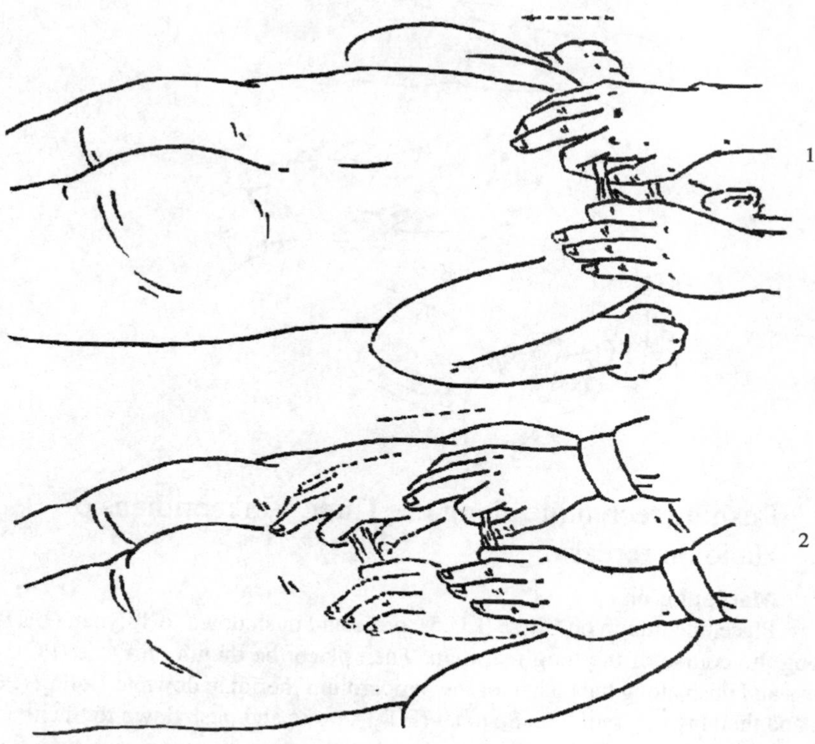

Holding and lifting techniques on the back.

Manipulation

Use two thumbs and index fingers to pinch Dazhu (BL 11) then keep on pinching and pulling up the muscle down the back past Pishu (BL 20) and stop at Guanyuanshu (BL 26). Repeat the manipulation for 3-5 times.

Points

1. Dazhu (BL 11): At the level of the lower border of the spinous process of the first thoracic vertebra and 1.5 *cun* lateral to the posterior midline.

2. Pishu (BL 20): At the level of the lower border of the spinous process of the eleventh thoracic vertebra and 1.5 *cun* lateral to the posterior midline.

3. Guanyuanshu (BL 26): At the level of the lower border of the spinous process of the fifth lumbar vertebra and 1.5 *cun* lateral to the posterior midline.

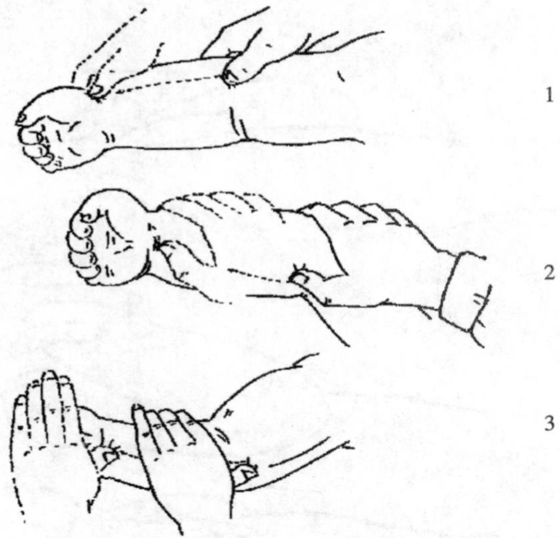

Pushing technique along the Three Yin meridians of Hand on forearm.

Manipulation

Place one thumb on Chize (LU 5), press and push down to Taiyuan (LU 9) along the course of the lung meridian. Then place the thumb on Quze (PC 3), press and push along the course of the pericardium meridian down to Daling (PC 7), and then lay the thumb on Shaohai (HT 3), press and push down to Shenmen (HT 7) following the heart meridian. Repeat the manipulation on each meridian for 1-2 minutes.

Points

1. Chize (LU 5): On the cubital crease, on the radial side of the tendon of m. biceps brachii. (He-sea point).

2. Taiyuan (LU 9): At the radial end of the transverse crease of the wrist, in the depression on the lateral side of the radial artery. (Shu-stream point).

3. Quze (PC 3): On the transverse cubital crease, at the ulnar side of the tendon of m. biceps brachii. (He-sea point).

4. Daling (PC 7): In the middle of the transverse crease of the wrist, between the tendons of m. palmaris longus and m. flexor carpi radialis. (Shu-stream point).

5. Shaohai (HT 3): When the elbow is flexed, the point is in the depression between the medial end of the transverse cubital crease and the medial epicondyle of the humerus.

6. Shenmen (HT 7): At the ulnar end of the transverse crease of the wrist, in the depression on the radial side of the tendon of m. flexor carpi ulnaris.

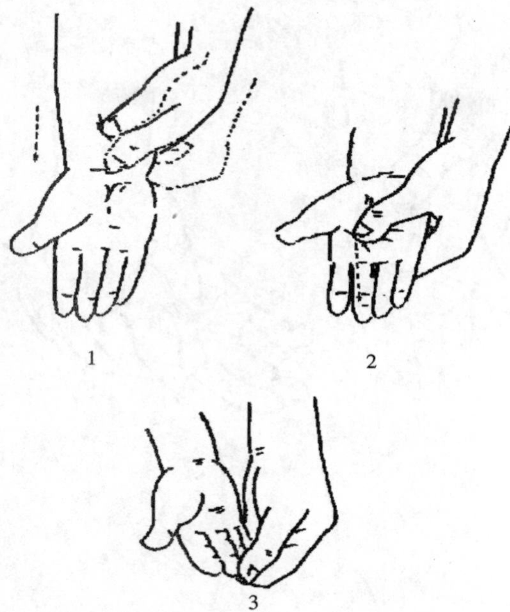

Opposite pressing technique on Waiguan (TE 5) and Neiguan (PC 6).

Manipulation

Place one thumb tip on Neiguan (PC 6) and other four fingertips on Waiguan (TE 5). Press the two points for 1-2 minutes, then press and push downwards past Daling (PC 7) and Yangchi (TE 4) to Laogong (PC 8) and Zhongchong (PC 9). Knead and press the points respectively for 1-2 minutes. Repeat the manipulation for 1-3 times.

Points

1. Neiguan (PC 6): 2 *cun* above the transverse crease of the wrist, between the tendons of m. palmaris longus and m. flexor radialis.
2. Waiguan (TE 5): 2 *cun* above the transverse crease of the dorsum of wrist, between the radius and ulna.
3. Daling (PC 7): In the middle of the transverse crease of the wrist, between the tendons of m. palmaris longus and m. flexor carpi radialis.
4. Yangchi (TE 4): On the transverse crease of the dorsum of wrist, in the depression lateral to the tendon of m. extensor digitorum communis.
5. Laogong (PC 8): On the transverse crease of the palm, between the second and third metacarpal bones.
6. Zhongchong (PC 9): In the center of the tip of the middle finger.

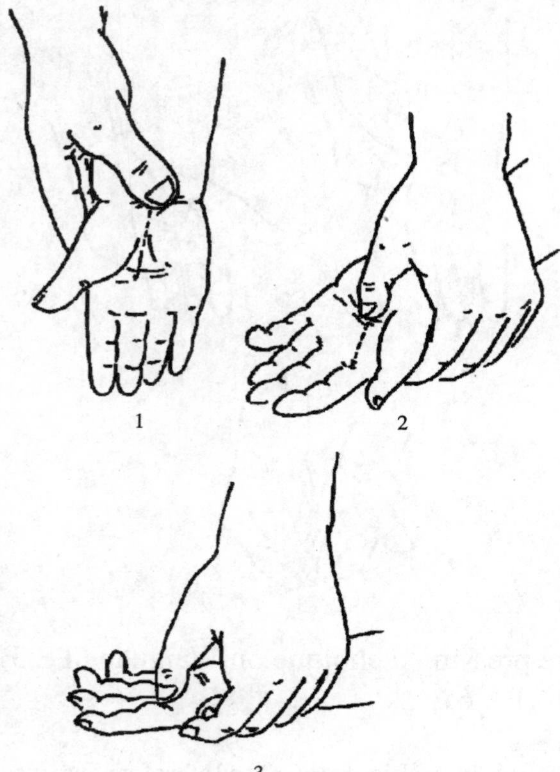

Stationary circular pressing technique on Laogong (PC 8).

Manipulation

Place one thumb on Daling (PC 7) and other four finger-pulps on the back of the wrist. From Daling (PC 7), press downwards to Laogong (PC 8), and knead Laogong (PC 8) with the thumb tip for 1-2 minutes, then push down to the proximal end of the index finger. Repeat the manipulation for 3-5 times.

Points

1. Daling (PC 7): In the middle of the transverse crease of the wrist, between the tendons of m. palmaris longus and m. flexor carpi radialis.

2. Laogong (PC 8): On the transverse crease of the palm, between the second and third metacarpal bones.

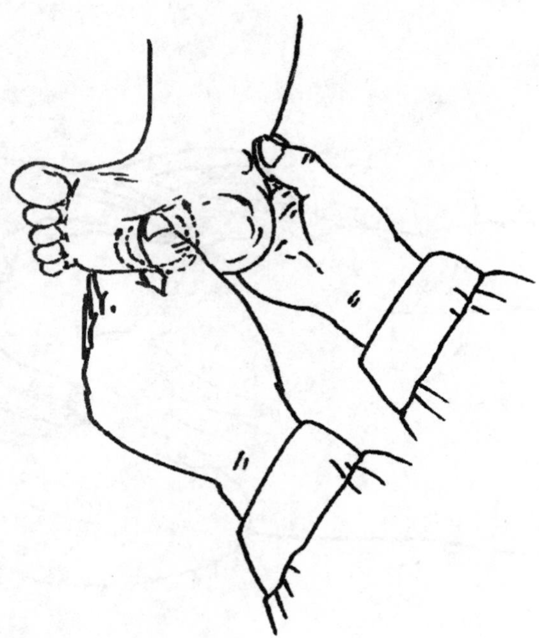

Stationary circular pressing technique on Yongquan (KI 1).

Manipulation

Use one hand to grab and press Achilles' tendon and place the thumb of the other hand on Yongquan (KI 1) located at the bottom of the foot, knead the point clockwise and counterclockwise. Make 50 circles of kneading in each direction.

Points

Yongquan (KI 1): On the sole, in the depression when the foot is in plantar flexion, approximately at the junction of the anterior one third and posterior two thirds of the sole.

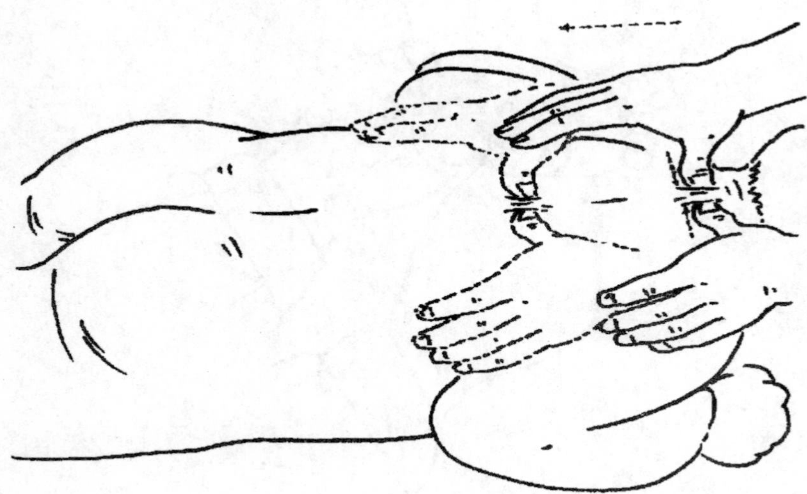

Squeezing and pushing techniques on the back.

Manipulation

With other fingers fanning out on each side of the back, place two thumb-pulps respectively on Dazhu (BL 11), squeeze and push the back muscle along the spine, and stop at Geshu (BL 17). Repeat the manipulation for 3-5 minutes.

Points

1. Dazhu (BL 11): At the level of the lower border of the spinous process of the first thoracic vertebra and 1.5 *cun* lateral to the midline.

2. Geshu (BL 17): At the level of the lower border of the spinous process of the seventh thoracic vertebra and 1.5 *cun* lateral to the midline.

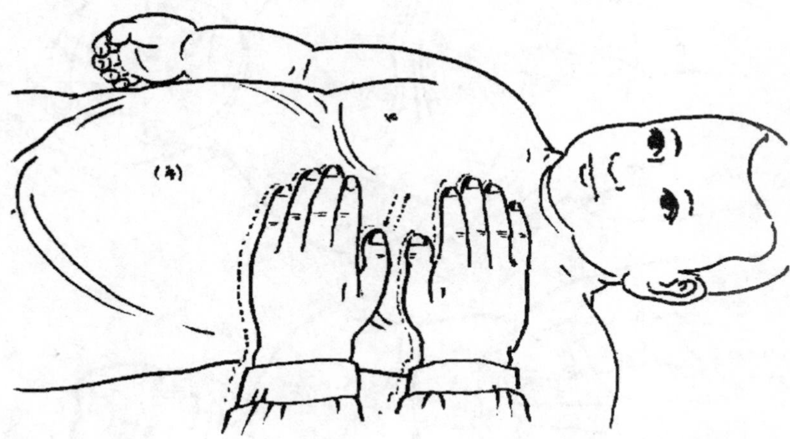

Chest extending technique.

Manipulation

Place two palm centres respectively on unilateral Yuanye (GB 22) and Dabao (SP 21) and the two thumb tips on Tianchi (PC 1) and Shidou (SP 17). Shake and press the points for 1-2 minutes.

Points

1. Yuanye (GB 22): On the mid-axillary line, in the fourth intercostal space.
2. Dabao (SP 21): On the mid-axillary line, in the sixth intercostal space.
3. Tianchi (PC 1): In the fourth intercostal space, 1 *cun* lateral to the nipple.
4. Shidou (SP 17): In the fifth intercostal space, 6 *cun* lateral to the anterior midline.

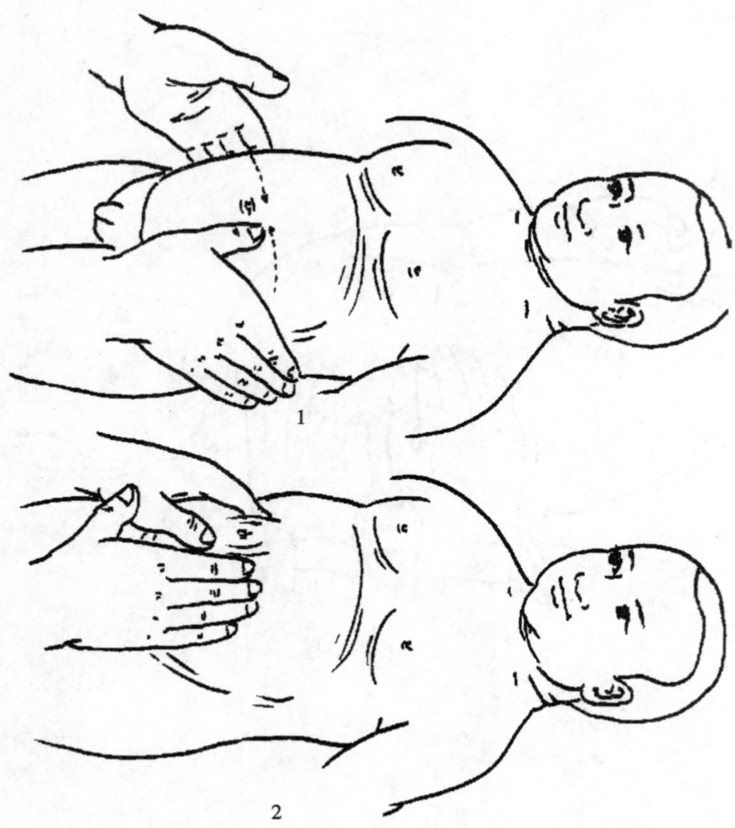

Squeezing and pushing techniques on the abdomen.

Manipulation

Place four finger-pulps of both hands respectively on bilateral Zhangmen (LR 13) and Jingmen (GB 25), then squeeze and rub towards the middle of the abdomen. Repeat the manipulation for 2-3 minutes.

Points

1. Zhangmen (LR 13): On the lateral side of the abdomen, below the free end of the eleventh floating rib.

2. Jingmen (GB 25): On the lateral side of the abdomen, below the free end of the twelfth floating rib.

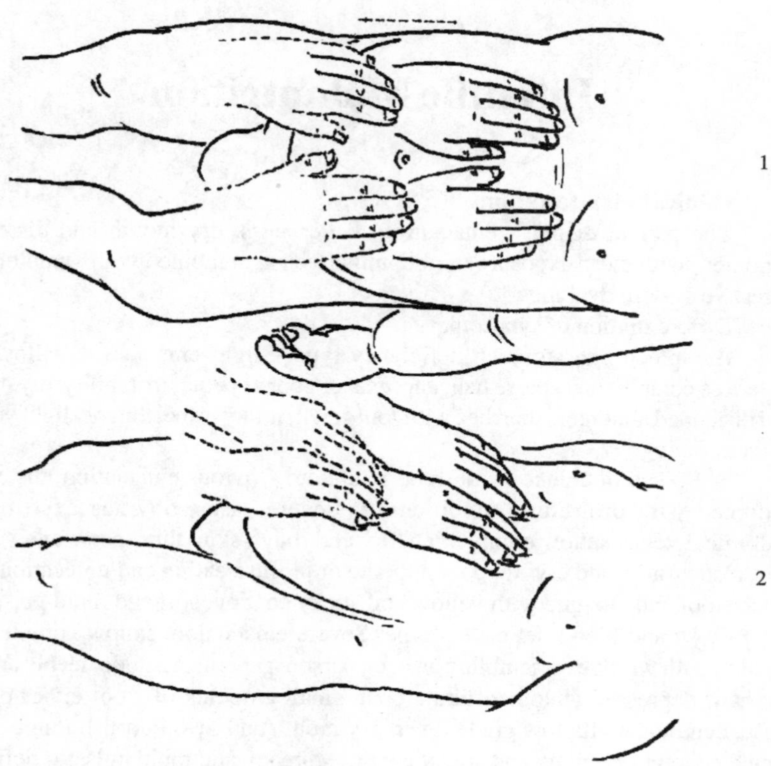

Rubbing and pressing techniques on the upper abdomen.

Manipulation

Place four finger-pulps of both hands on Burong (ST 19) and rub downwards to Tianshu (ST 25). Repeat the massage for 1-2 minutes, then press Burong (ST 19) and Tianshu (ST 25) for 1-2 minutes.

Points

1. Burong (ST 19): 6 *cun* above the umbilicus and 2 *cun* lateral to the midline.
2. Tianshu (ST 25): 2 *cun* lateral to the center of the umbilicus.

Infantile Malnutrition

Clinical Manifestations

The patient displays emaciation, listlessness, dry mouth and distended abdomen, with clear exposure of abdominal veins, combined with symptoms of digestive system dysfunction.

Differentiation of syndromes:

A. Spleen and stomach deficiency type: Slight emaciation, sallow and lusterless complexion, sparse hair, anorexia or poor appetite, irritability, dry mouth and distended abdomen, diarrhea with foul smell, milky urine, thin or slight yellow tongue coating.

B. Spleen deficiency with food retention: Obvious emaciation, distended abdomen with protruding umbilicus; in severe cases, obvious exposure of abdominal veins, sallow complexion, dry and rough skin, thin sparse and yellow hair, restlessness and crying, poor appetite or profuse eating and defecation with much stool, pale tongue with yellow and sticky coating, soft and rapid pulse.

C. *Qi* and blood deficiency type: Severe emaciation, sallow complexion, dry skin with wrinkles resembling an aged person, general lassitude, feeble crying, dry hair, depressed abdomen like a boat, small amounts of stool either dry or loose, combined with low grade fever, dry mouth and lips. Purplish tongue with peeled coating or yellow and sticky coating, thready and rapid pulse or deficient type of pulse.

Treatment Principle

Regulating the spleen and stomach, dispelling the pathogenic factors.

Tuina Techniques

A. Circular kneading technique on periumbilical region.
B. Transverse rubbing technique on the upper abdomen.
C. Pressing technique on Tianshu (ST 25).
D. Holding and lifting techniques of the abdominal muscles.
E. Digital pressing technique on the hypochondrium for reinforcing *qi*.
F. Straight rubbing technique on the back.
G. Holding and lifting technique on the back.

H. Stationary circular kneading technique on Mingmen (GV 4).

Addition or Subtraction Techniques

A. Spleen and stomach deficiency type:

Addition: 1. Stationary circular kneading technique on Zusanli (ST 36). 2. Stationary circular kneading technique on Neiguan (PC 6) and Waiguan (TE 5).

B. Spleen deficiency with food retention:

Addition: Transverse rubbing technique across the umbilicus.

Subtraction: 1. Holding and lifting techniques of the abdominal muscles. 2. Digital pressing technique on the hypochondrium for reinforcing *qi*.

A. *Qi* and blood deficiency type:

Addition: 1. Stationary circular kneading technique on Sanyinjiao (SP 6). 2. Nipping technique on Sishencong (Ex-HN 1).

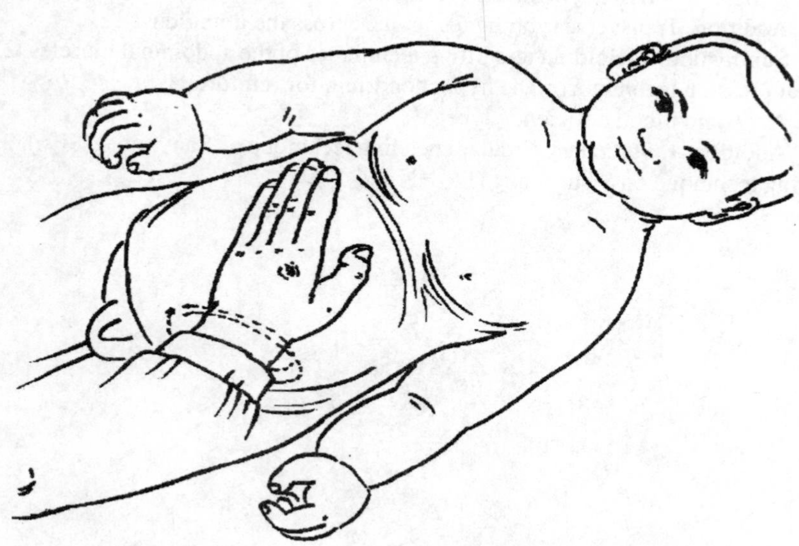

Circular kneading technique on periumbilical region.

Manipulation

Lay the center of a palm on Shenque (CV 8), knead the point clockwise and counterclockwise in each direction, the massage should last 2-3 minutes.

Points

Shenque (CV 8): In the center of the umbilicus.

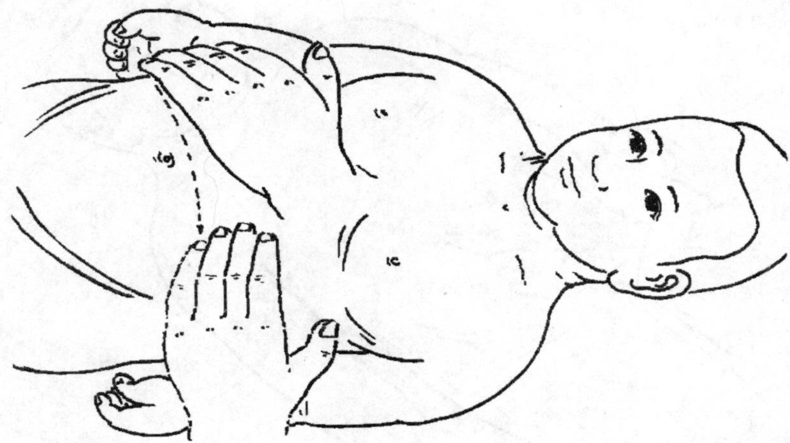

Transverse rubbing technique on the upper abdomen.

Manipulation

Place one palm on Fuai (SP 16) and Daheng (SP 15) on one side, rub transversely across the abdomen to Fuai (SP 16) and Daheng (SP 15) on the other side. Repeat the manipulation for 5-10 minutes.

Points

1. Fuai (SP 16): 4 *cun* directly above the center of the umbilicus and 4 *cun* lateral to the midline.

2. Daheng (SP 15): 4 *cun* lateral to the center of the umbilicus.

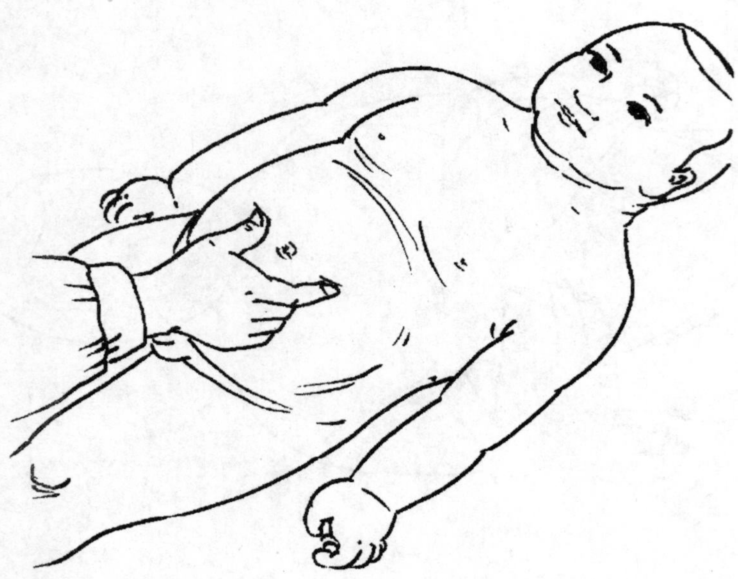

Pressing technique on Tianshu (ST 25).

Manipulation

Place the thumb tip and index finger tip of one hand respectively on bilateral Tianshu (ST 25), press and knead the points forcefully for 3-5 times, each time should last 1-2 minutes.

Points

Tianshu (ST 25): 2 *cun* lateral to the center of the umbilicus.

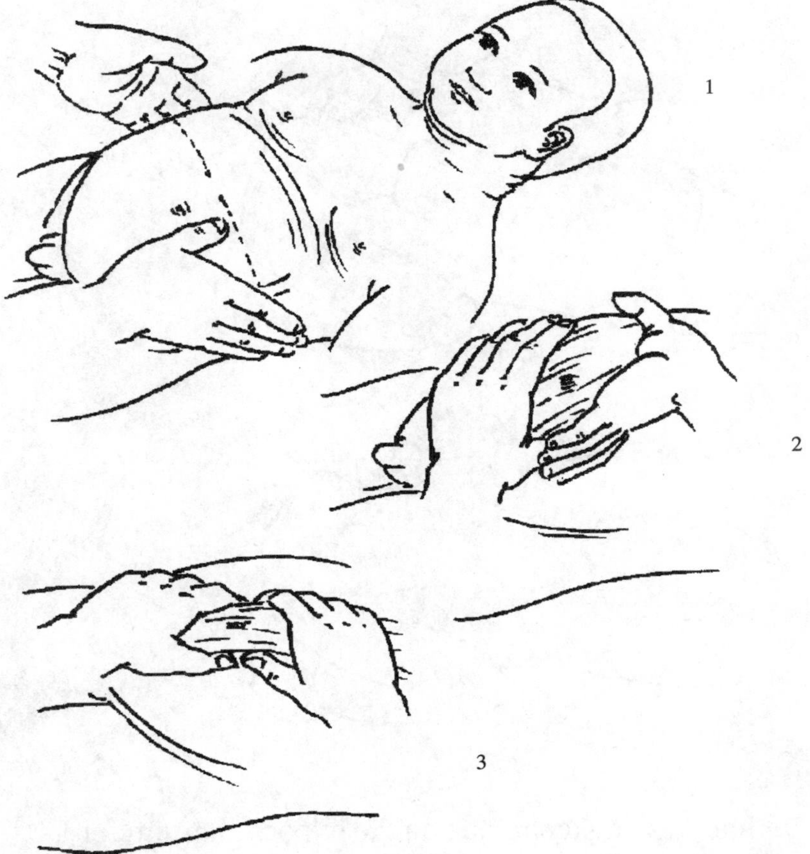

Holding and lifting techniques on the abdominal muscles.

Manipulation

Place respectively the four finger-pulps of both hands on bilateral Zhangmen (LR 13), squeeze and push vigorously the abdominal muscles towards the middle of the abdomen. Turn one hand, let the other hand keep on pushing the muscle, then both hands grasp and lift the squeezed abdominal muscle at the middle of the abdomen 3-5 times, (see fig.3). Each time lasts 5-10 seconds.

Points

Zhangmen (LR 13): On the lateral side of the abdomen, below the free end of the eleventh floating rib.

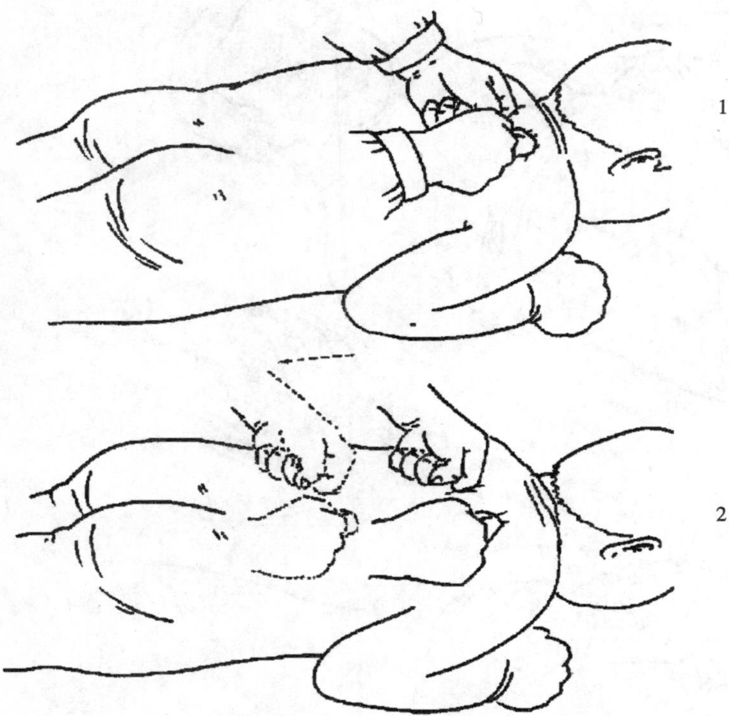

Digital pressing technique on the hypochondrium for reinforcing *qi*.

Manipulation

Place the index finger knuckles of both hands respectively on bilateral Dazhu (BL 11) then press straight downwards along the first line of Bladder Meridian, pass Xinshu (BL 15) and stop at Geshu (BL 17). Repeat the manipulation for 3-5 times.

Points

1. Dazhu (BL 11): At the level of the lower border of the spinous process of the first thoracic vertebra and 1.5 *cun* lateral to the posterior midline.

2. Xinshu (BL 15): At the level of the lower border of the spinous process of the fifth thoracic vertebra and 1.5 *cun* lateral to the posterior midline.

3. Geshu (BL 17): At the level of the lower border of the spinous process of the seventh thoracic vertebra and 1.5 *cun* lateral to the posterior midline.

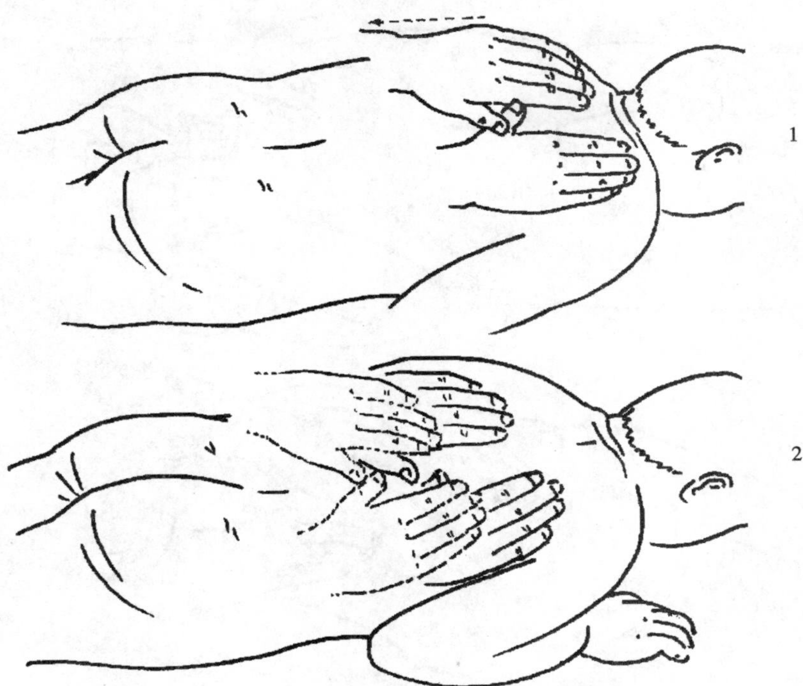

Straight rubbing technique on the back.

Manipulation

Place four finger-pulps of both hands on Dazhu (BL 11), rub straight downwards along both sides of the spine past Jueyinshu (BL 14) and stop at Geshu (BL 17). Knead the acupoints located along the massage region one by one. Repeat the manipulation for 3-5 minutes.

Points

1. Dazhu (BL 11): At the level of the lower border of the spinous process of the first thoracic vertebra and 1.5 *cun* lateral to the midline.

2. Jueyinshu (BL 14): At the level of the lower border of the spinous process of the fourth thoracic vertebra and 1.5 *cun* lateral to the midline.

3. Geshu (BL 17):. At the level of the lower border of the spinous process of the seventh thoracic vertebra and 1.5 *cun* lateral to the midline.

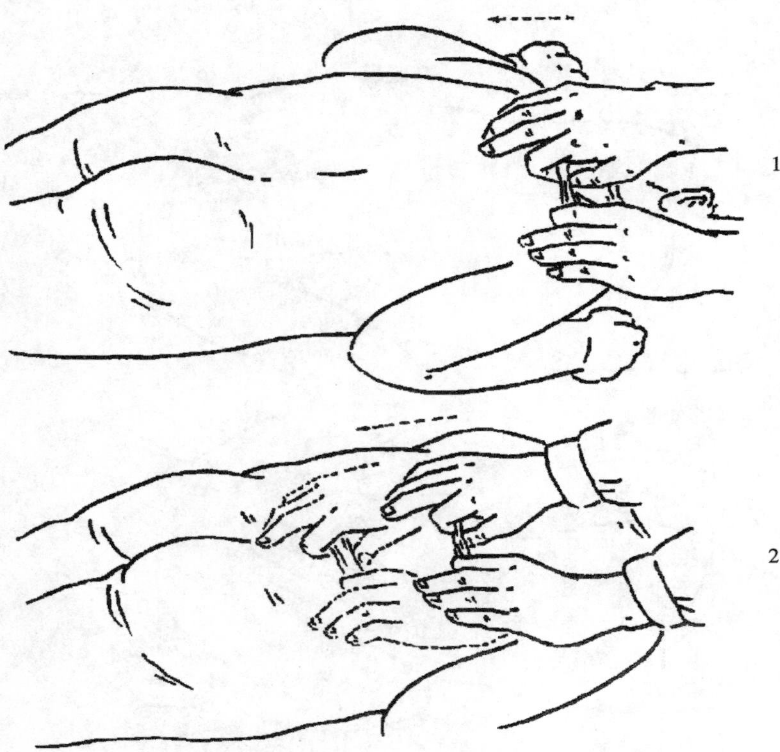

Holding and lifting techniques on the back.

Manipulation

Use two thumbs and index fingers of both hands to pinch Dazhu (BL 11) then keep on pinching and pulling up the muscle down the back past Pishu (BL 20) and stop at Guanyuanshu (BL 26). Repeat the manipulation for 3-5 times.

Points

1. Dazhu (BL 11): At the level of the lower border of the spinous process of the first thoracic vertebra and 1.5 *cun* lateral to the posterior midline.

2. Pishu (BL 20): At the level of the lower border of the spinous process of the eleventh thoracic vertebra and 1.5 *cun* lateral to the posterior midline.

3. Guanyuanshu (BL 26): At the level of the lower border of the spinous process of the fifth lumbar vertebra and 1.5 *cun* lateral to the posterior midline.

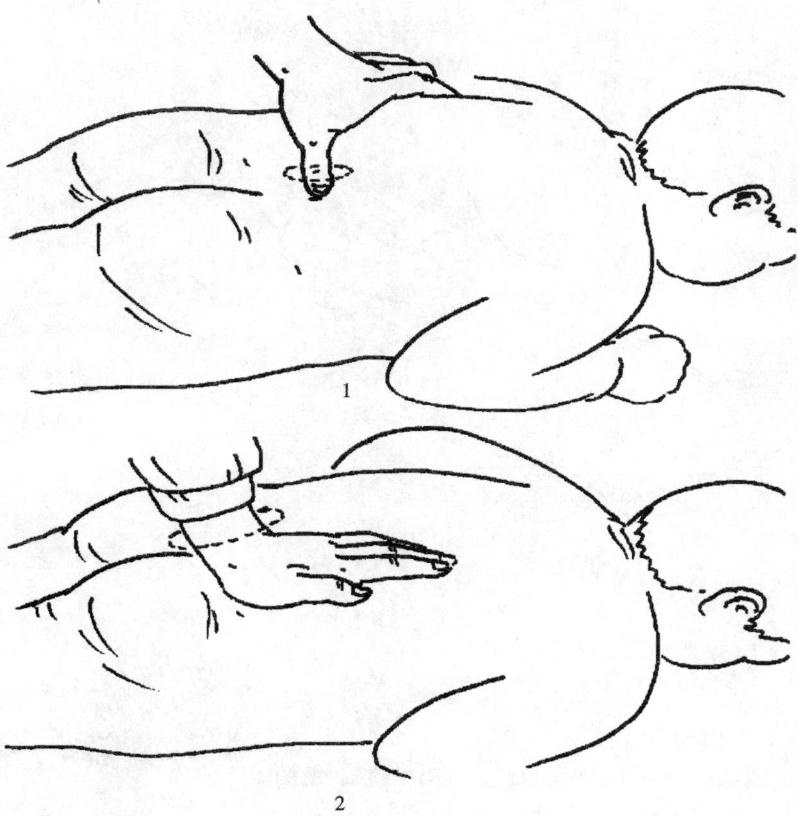

Stationary circular pressing technique on Mingmen (GV 4).

Manipulation

Place a thumb on Mingmen (GV 4), press and knead the point for 2-3 minutes, then place the palm flat on the same area and conduct circular pressing with the palm as shown in figure 2 for 1-2 minutes.

Points

Mingmen (GV 4): Below the spinous process of the second lumbar vertebra.

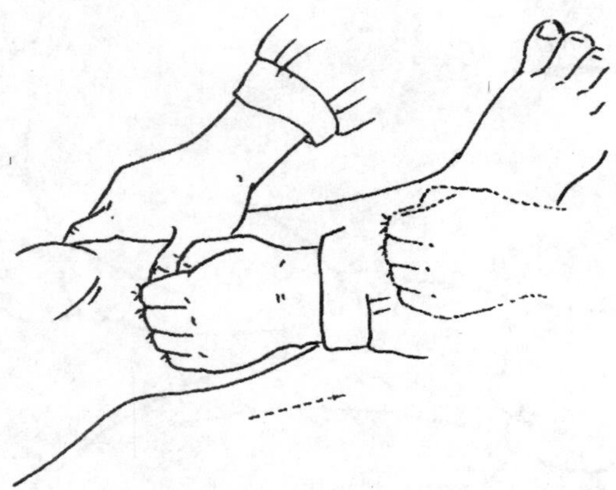

Stationary circular pressing technique on Zusanli (ST 36).

Manipulation

Place a thumb on Zusanli (ST 36) and press the point. At the same time, flex four fingers of the other hand and place them on Yanglingquan (GB 34), and push downwards to Xuanzhong (GB 39). Repeat the manipulation for 1-2 minutes.

Points

1. Zusanli (ST 36): One finger-breadth lateral to the anterior crest of the tibia, in m. tibialis anterior.

2. Yanglingquan (GB 34): In the depression anterior and inferior to the head of the fibula.

3. Xuanzhong (GB 39): 3 *cun* above the tip of the external malleolus, in the depression between the posterior border of the fibula and the tendons of m. peroneus longus and brevis.

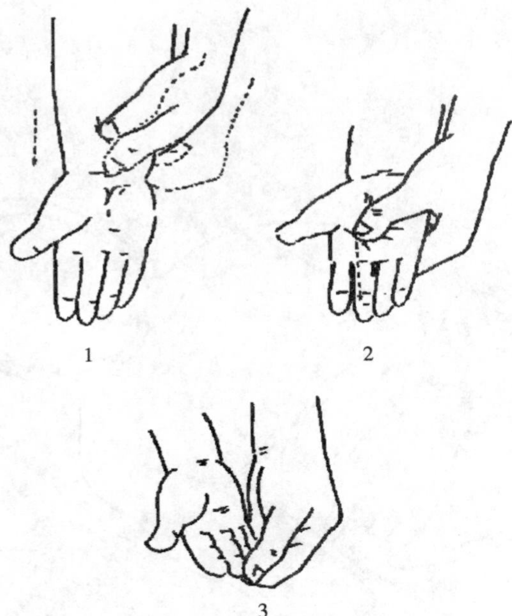

Opposite pressing technique on Waiguan (TE 5) and Neiguan (PC 6).

Manipulation

Place one thumb tip on Neiguan (PC 6) and other four fingertips on Waiguan (TE 5). Press the two points for 1-2 minutes, then press and push downwards past Daling (PC 7) and Yangchi (TE 4) to Laogong (PC 8) and Zhongchong (PC 9). Knead each point respectively for 1-2 minutes. Repeat the manipulation for 1-3 times.

Points

1. Neiguan (PC 6): 2 *cun* above the transverse crease of the wrist, between the tendons of m. palmaris longus and m. flexor radialis.

2. Waiguan (TE 5): 2 *cun* above the transverse crease of the dorsum of wrist, between the radius and ulna.

3. Daling (PC 7): In the middle of the transverse crease of the wrist, between the tendons of m. palmaris longus and m. flexor carpi radialis.

4. Yangchi (TE 4): On the transverse crease of the dorsum of wrist, in the depression lateral to the tendon of m. extensor digitorum communis.

5. Laogong (PC 8): On the transverse crease of the palm, between the second and third metacarpal bones.

6. Zhongchong (PC 9): In the center of the tip of the middle finger.

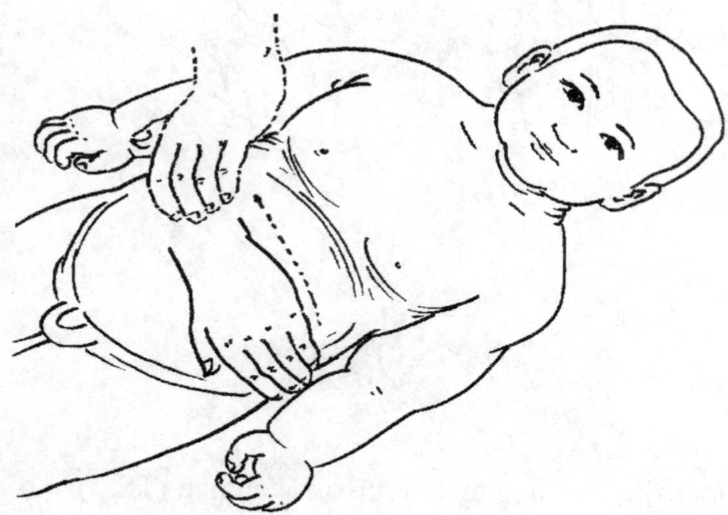

Transverse rubbing technique across the umbilicus.

Manipulation

Place four finger-pulps on one side of Daheng (SP 15) and Fujie (SP 14), rub transversely across the abdomen and past Tianshu (ST 25) and Wailing (ST 26), stop at Daheng (SP 15) and Fujie (SP 14) on the opposite. Repeat the manipulation for 2-3 minutes.

Points

1. Daheng (SP 15): 4 *cun* lateral to the center of the umbilicus.
2. Fujie (SP 14): 1.3 *cun* below the umbilicus and 4 *cun* lateral to the midline.
3. Tianshu (ST 25): 2 *cun* lateral to the center of the umbilicus.
4. Wailing (ST 26): 1 *cun* below the center of the umbilicus and 2 *cun* lateral to the midline.

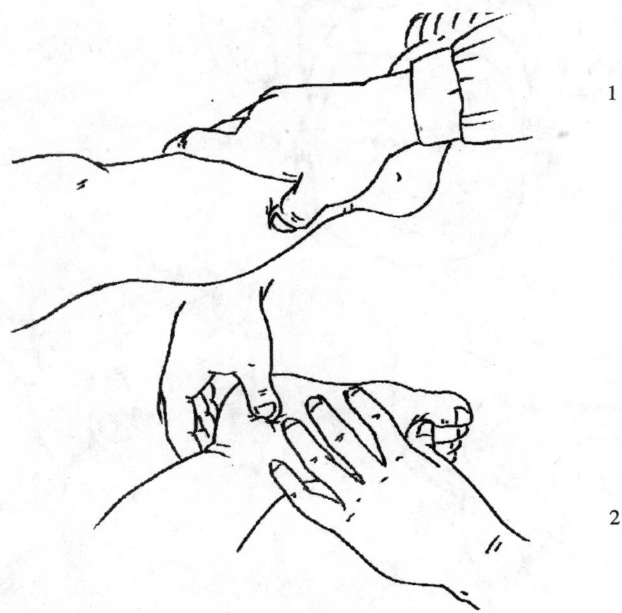

Stationary circular pressing technique on Sanyinjiao (SP 6).

Manipulation

Place a thumb tip on Sanyinjiao (SP 6), press and knead the point for 2-5 minutes. Then move the thumb tip to Zhaohai (KI 6), meanwhile place the other thumb tip on Taichong (LR 3), press and knead the two points at the same time for 1-3 minutes.

Points

1. Sanyinjiao (SP 6): 3 *cun* directly above the tip of the medial malleolus, on the posterior border of the medial aspect of the tibia.

2. Zhaohai (KI 6): In the depression of the lower border of the medial malleolus.

3. Taichong (LR 3): On the dorsum of the foot, in the depression distal to the junction of the first and second metatarsal bones.

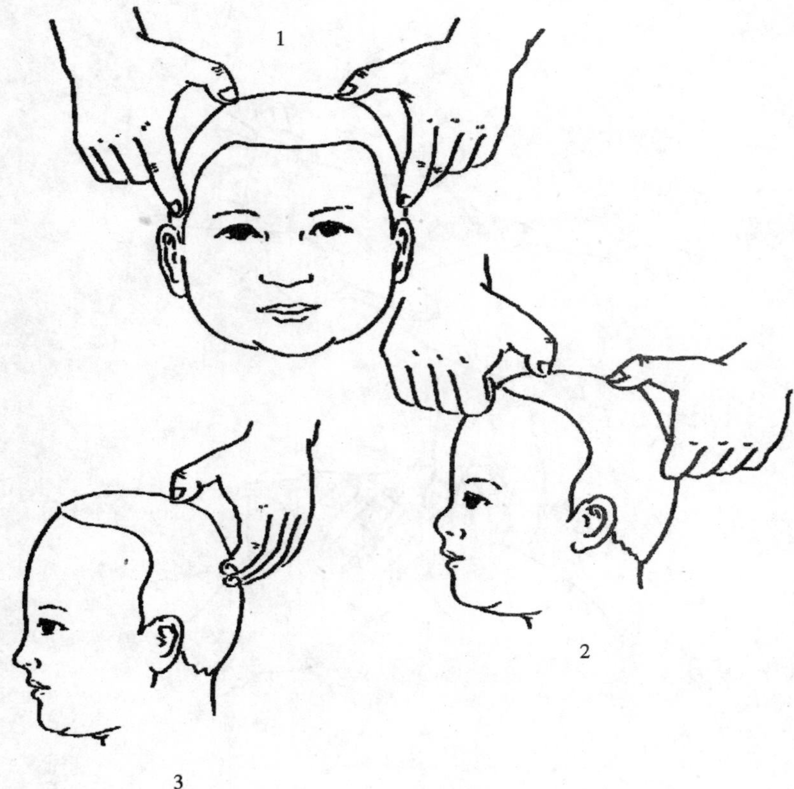

Nipping technique on Sishencong (Ex-HN 1)

Manipulation

Place two thumb tips on bilateral Luoque (BL 18), nip (press sharply) the points first, and knead them next. Then apply the same massage on Qianding (GV 21) and Houding (GV 19). Lastly massage Baihui (GV 20) in the same way. Repeat the manipulation for 2-3 minutes.

Points

1. Luoque (BL 8): 5.5 *cun* directly above midpoint of the anterior hairline and 1.5 *cun* lateral to the midline.
2. Qianding (GV 21): 3.5 *cun* directly above the middle of the anterior hairline.
3. Houding (GV 19): 6.5 *cun* directly above the middle of the anterior hairline.
4. Baihui (GV 20): 5 *cun* directly above the middle of the anterior hairline.

Dysmenorrhea

Clinical Manifestations

Before, during or after menstruation, there is pain in the lower abdomen, which may radiate to the lumbar and sacrum region, or even result in syncopy in severe cases. Acute surgical abdomen disease should be excluded.

Differentiation of syndromes:

A. *Qi* obstruction and blood stagnation type: Distending pain with dislike of pressure occurring during or 1-2 days before menstruation, less menstrual flow in quantity and dark purplish in color with clots; the pain being reduced after removal of the clots; purplish tongue with wiry and tense pulse.

B. Cold retention and *qi* obstruction type: Cold pain in the lower abdomen relieved by warmth and aggravated by pressure, menstrual flow less in quantity and dark black in color with clots, white and sticky coating, deep and tense pulse.

C. *Qi* and blood deficiency type: Dull pain in the lower abdomen appearing during or 1-2 days after menstruation, menstrual flow less in quantity, light in color and thin in quality, combined with empty and bearing down sensation in the lower abdomen and the pubic region, preference of pressure on the abdomen, general lassitude, poor appetite and diarrhea, pale tongue with thin and sticky coating, thready pulse.

D. Liver and kidney Yin deficiency type: Lingering dull pain in the lower abdomen 1-2 days after menstruation, menstrual flow less in quantity, light dark in color and thin in quality, combined with soreness in the lumbar region, afternoon fever, tinnitus, constipation and irritability, red tongue with thin coating or no coating, thready and rapid pulse.

Treatment Principle

Regulating menstruation and relieving pain.

Tuina Techniques

A. Transverse rubbing technique on the upper abdomen.

B. Transverse rubbing technique on the superior border of the pubis.

C. Pressing technique along the medial border of the iliac bone.

D. Rubbing chest technique.

E. Kneading and pinching techniques along the medial aspect of the thigh.
F. Squeezing and pushing techniques on the back.
G. Lateral thumb pushing technique on the lumbar region.

Addition or Subtraction Techniques

A. *Qi* obstruction and blood stagnation type:

Addition: Big relieving *qi* stagnation technique.

B. Cold retention and *qi* obstruction type:

Addition: 1. Rubbing technique on the sides of the umbilicus. 2. Pressing technique on *Qi*chong (ST 30). 3. Stationary circular pressing technique on Sanyinjiao (SP 6).

C. *Qi* and blood deficiency type:

Addition: Pushing technique on the side of the abdomen. 2. Digital pressing technique on the hypochondrium for reinforcing *qi*.

Subtraction: Rubbing chest technique.

D. Liver and kidney Yin deficiency type:

Addition: 1. Kneading technique on the lumbosacral region. 2. Diagonal rubbing technique on the sacrum. 3. Overlapping palm pressing technique on the lumbar region.

Subtraction: Rubbing chest technique.

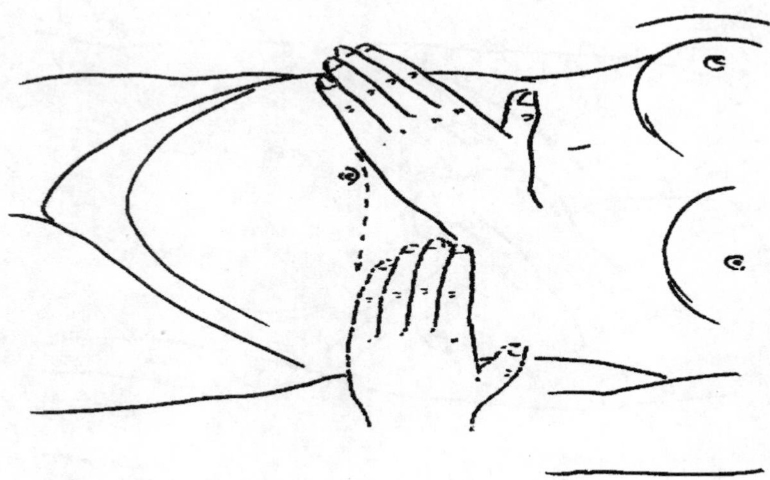

Transverse rubbing technique on the upper abdomen.

Manipulation

Place one palm on Fuai (SP 16) and Daheng (SP 15) of one side, rub transversely across the abdomen to Fuai (SP 16) and Daheng (SP 15) on the other side. Repeat the manipulation for 5-10 minutes.

Points

1. Fuai (SP 16): 4 *cun* directly above the center of the umbilicus and 4 *cun* lateral to the midline.

2. Daheng (SP 15): 4 *cun* lateral to the center of the umbilicus.

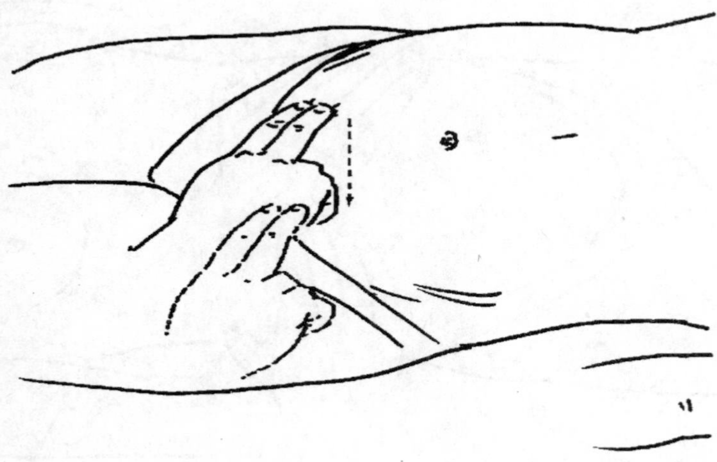

Transverse rubbing technique on the superior border of the pubis.

Manipulation

Place the index and middle finger-pulps of one hand on unilateral Guilai (ST 29) and Qichong (ST 30), rub transversely across the abdomen (above the pubic bone) to the opposite Guilai (ST 29) and Qichong (ST 30). Repeat the manipulation for 5-10 minutes.

Points

1. Guilai (ST 29): 4 *cun* directly below the center of the umbilicus and 2 *cun* lateral to the midline.

2. Qichong (ST 30): 1 *cun* directly below Guilai (ST 29).

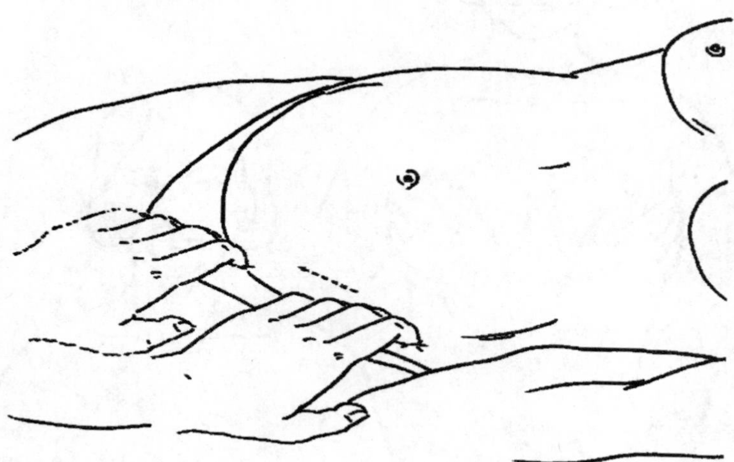

Pressing technique along the medial border of the iliac bone.

Manipulation

Place four fingertips on Wushu (GB 27) on the side of the ilium, press and push down to Qichong (ST 30). Repeat the manipulation for 1-2 minutes.

Points

1. Wushu (GB 27): 0.5 *cun* anterior to the anterior superior iliac spine.
2. Qichong (ST 30): 5 *cun* directly below the center of the umbilicus and 2 *cun* lateral to the anterior midline.

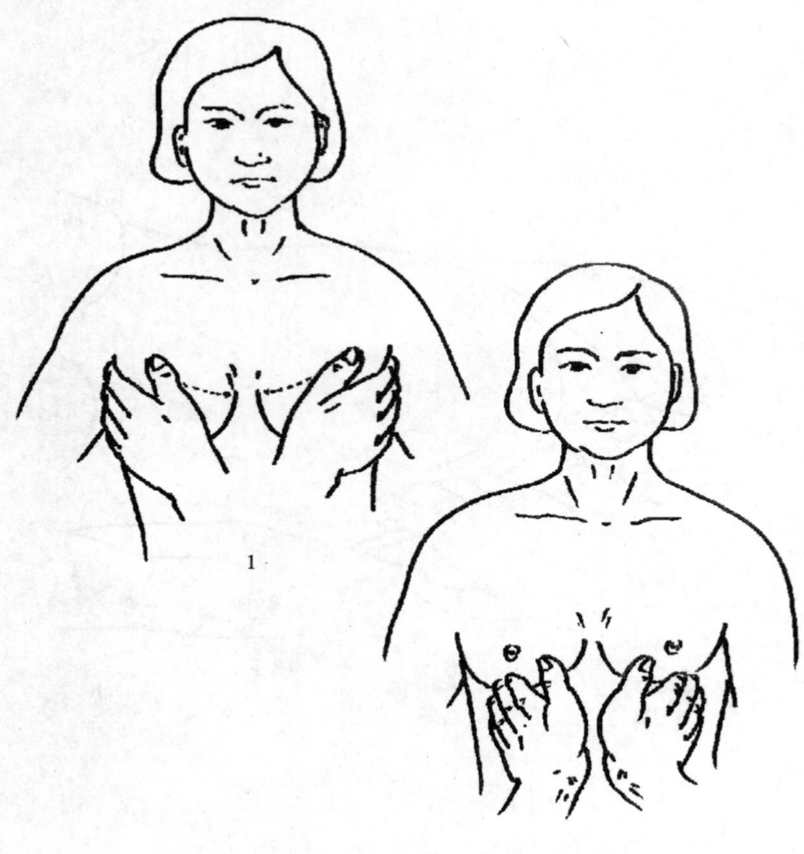

Rubbing chest technique.

Manipulation

Place two palms respectively on bilateral Yuanye (GB 22) and Dabao (SP 21) and the fingers on the intercostal spaces. Rub from Yuanye (GB 22) and Dabao (SP 21) located at the outside of the breasts to the middle, stop at Qimen (LR 14). Repeat the manipulation for 1-3 minutes.

Points

1. Yuanye (GB 22): On the mid-axillary line, in the fourth intercostal space.
2. Dabao (SP 21): On the mid-axillary line, in the sixth intercostal space.
3. Qimen (LR 14): Directly below the nipple, in the sixth intercostal space.

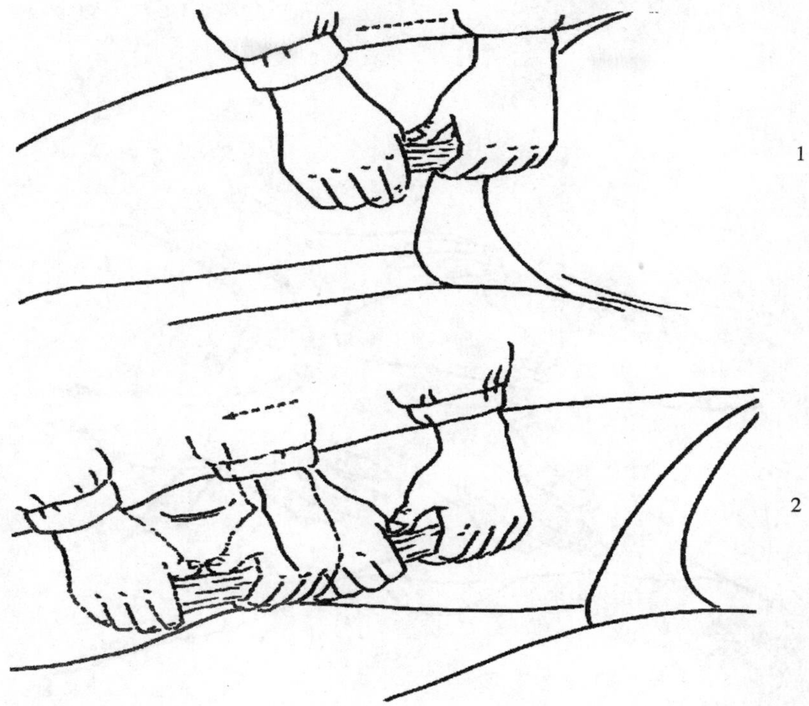

Kneading and pinching techniques along the medial aspect of the thigh.

Manipulation

Place fingertips of both hands on Yinlian (LR 11) and Zuwuli (LR 10), pinch and squeeze the medial thigh muscle from Yinbao (LR 9) to Ququan (LR 8). Repeat the manipulation for 3-5 minutes.

Points

1. Yinlian (LR 11): 2 *cun* lateral and 2 *cun* below the midpoint of the upper margin of the pubic bone.
2. Zuwuli (LR 10): 1 *cun* directly below Yinlian (LR 11).
3. Yinbao (LR 9): 4 *cun* above the medial epicondyle of the femur, at the posterior border of m. sartorius.
4. Ququan (LR 8): When the knee is flexed, the point is in the depression above the medial end of the transverse popliteal crease.

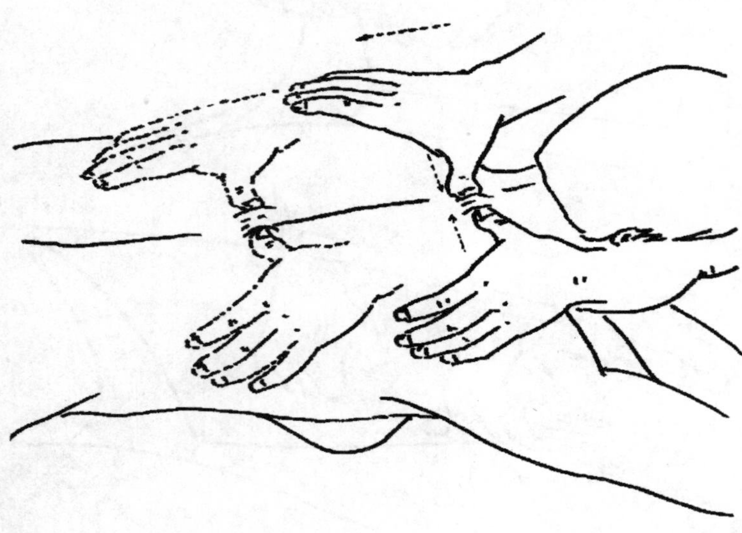

Squeezing and pushing techniques on the back.

Manipulation

With other fingers fanning out on each side of the back, place two thumb-pulps respectively on Dazhu (BL 11), squeeze and push the back muscle along the spine and stop at Geshu (BL 17). Repeat the manipulation for 3-5 minutes.

Points

1. Dazhu (BL 11): At the level of the lower border of the spinous process of the first thoracic vertebra and 1.5 *cun* lateral to the midline.

2. Geshu (BL 17): At the level of the lower border of the spinous process of the seventh thoracic vertebra and 1.5 *cun* lateral to the midline.

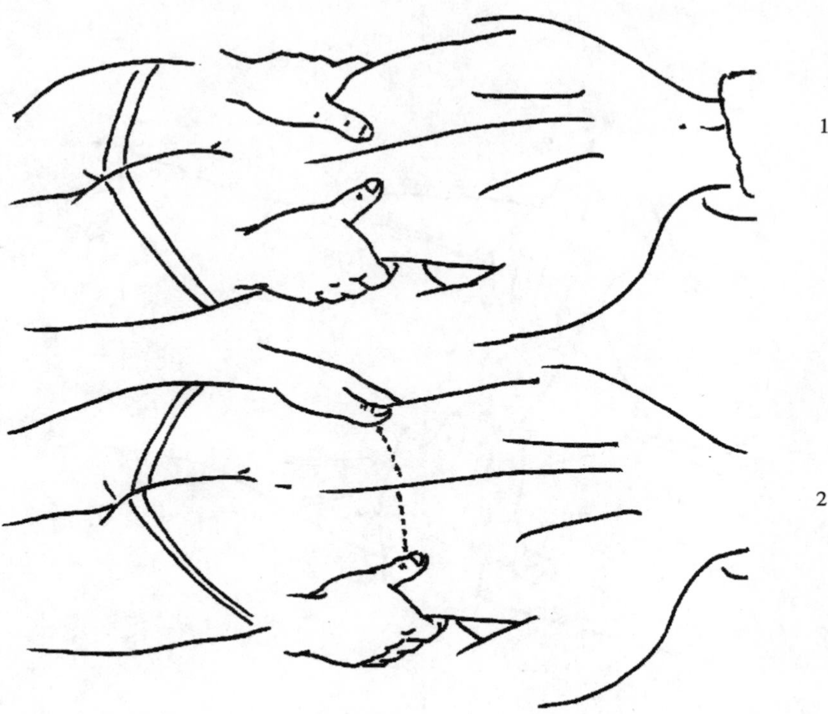

Lateral thumb pushing technique on the lumbar region.

Manipulation

Place two thumbs respectively on bilateral Shenshu (BL 23) and other four fingers around the waist, and conduct pushing technique at Shenshu (BL 23), move laterally from middle of the back to the side of the back, and stop at Daimai (GB 26). Repeat the manipulation for 1-3 minutes.

Points

1. Shenshu (BL 23): At the level of the lower border of the spinous process of the second lumbar vertebra and 1.5 *cun* lateral to the posterior midline.

2. Daimai (GB 26): Directly below the free end of the eleventh rib, at the level with the umbilicus.

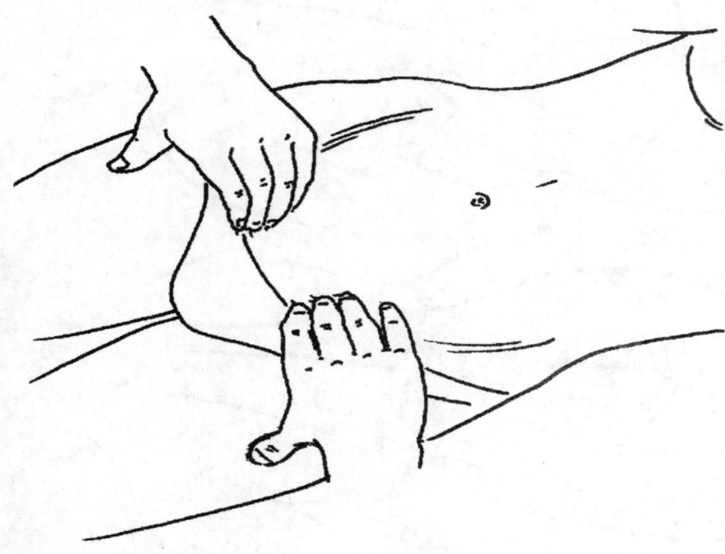

Big relieving *qi* stagnation technique.

Manipulation

Place four finger-pulps of both hands on bilateral Guilai (ST 29) and Qichong (ST 30) located at the lower abdomen. Press the points 1-3 times, each time should last 15-60 seconds.

Points

1. Guilai (ST 29): 4 *cun* below the center of the umbilicus and 2 *cun* lateral to the midline.

2. Qichong (ST 30): 5 *cun* below the center of the umbilicus and 2 *cun* lateral to the midline.

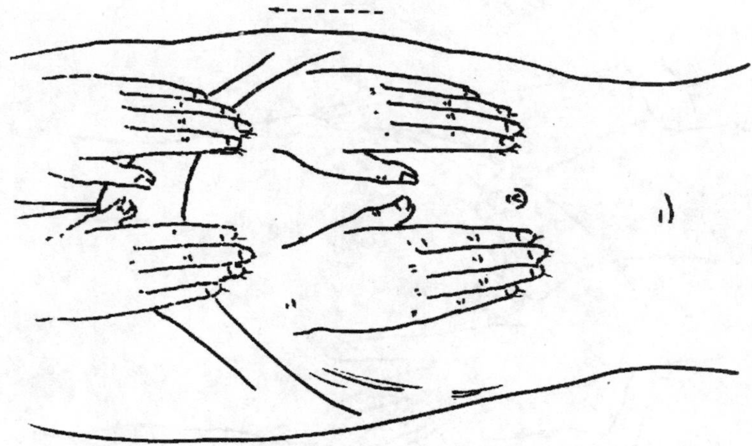

Rubbing technique on the sides of the umbilicus.

Manipulation

Place four finger-pulps of both hands on Tianshu (ST 25) and Huangshu (KI 16), then rub downwards to Shuidao (ST 28) and Qixue (KI 13). Repeat the manipulation for 5-10 minutes.

Points

1. Tianshu (ST 25): 2 *cun* lateral to the center of the umbilicus.
2. Huangshu (KI 16): 0.5 *cun* lateral to the center of the umbilicus.
3. Shuidao (ST 28): 3 *cun* directly below the center of the umbilicus and 2 *cun* lateral to the midline.
4. Qixue (KI 13): 3 *cun* directly below the center of the umbilicus and 0.5 *cun* lateral to the midline.

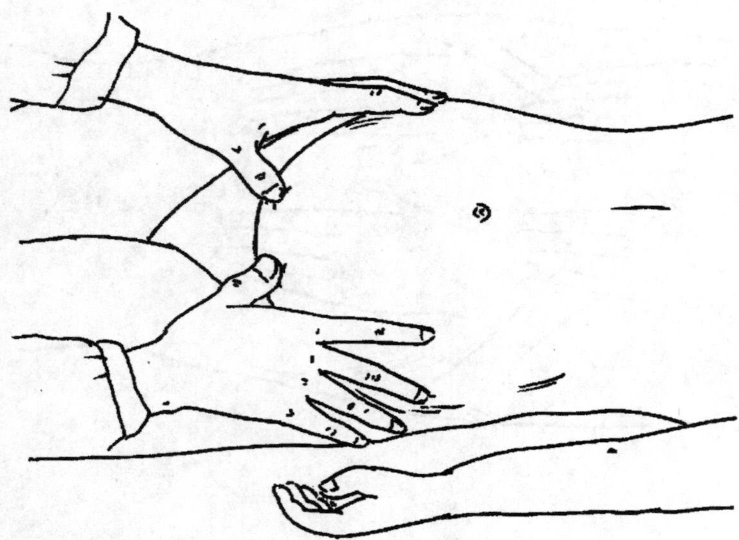

Pressing technique on Qichong (ST 30).

Manipulation

Place two thumbs on bilateral Qichong (ST 30) and press the points for 1-3 times, each time lasts 10-30 seconds, and then release the thumbs.

Points

Qichong (ST 30): 5 *cun* directly below the center of the umbilicus and 2 *cun* lateral to the midline.

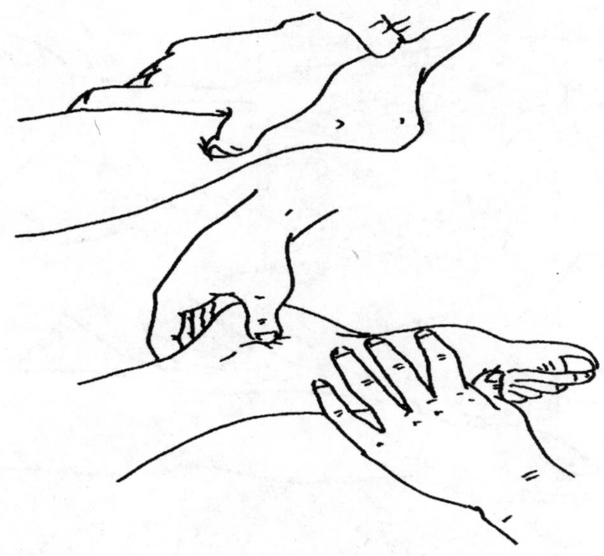

Stationary circular pressing technique on Sanyinjiao (SP 6).

Manipulation

Place a thumb tip on Sanyinjiao (SP 6), press and knead the point for 2-5 minutes. Then move the thumb tip to Zhaohai (KI 6), meanwhile place the other thumb tip on Taichong (LR 3), press and knead the two points at the same time for 1-3 minutes.

Points

1. Sanyinjiao (SP 6): 3 *cun* directly above the tip of the medial malleolus, on the posterior border of the medial aspect of the tibia.

2. Zhaohai (KI 6): In the depression of the lower border of the medial malleolus.

3. Taichong (LR 3): On the dorsum of the foot, in the depression distal to the junction of the first and second metatarsal bones.

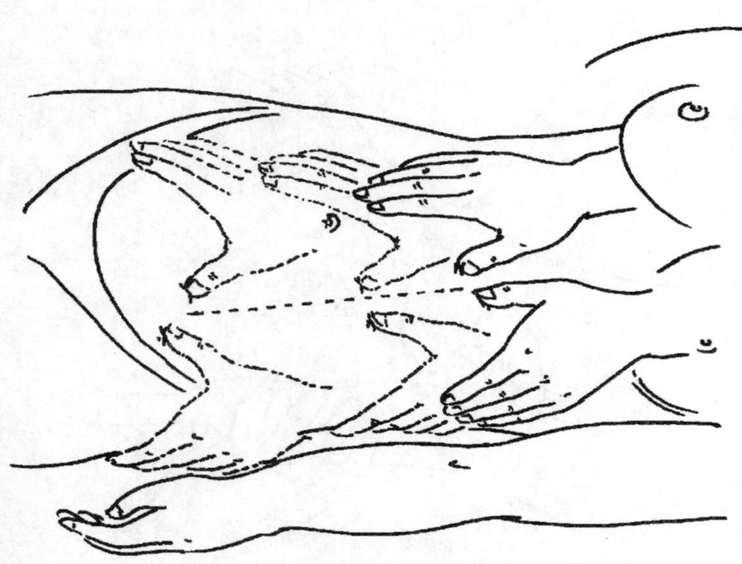

Pushing technique on the side of the abdomen.

Manipulation

Place two thumbs respectively on Fuai (SP 16) and Guanmen (ST 22) and other four fingers on the two sides of the stomach. Rub straight downwards past Daheng (SP 15) and Tianshu (ST 25) and stop at Fushe (SP 13) and Shuidao (ST 28). Repeat the manipulation for 2-3 minutes.

Points

1. Fuai (SP 16): 3 *cun* directly above the center of the umbilicus and 4 *cun* lateral to the midline.

2. Guanmen (ST 22): 3 *cun* directly above the center of the umbilicus and 2 *cun* lateral to the midline.

3. Daheng (SP 15): 4 *cun* lateral to the center of the umbilicus.

4. Tianshu (ST 25): 2 *cun* lateral to the center of the umbilicus.

5. Fushe (SP 13): 3.5 *cun* directly below the center of the umbilicus and 4 *cun* lateral to the midline.

6. Shuidao (ST 28): 3 *cun* directly below the center of the umbilicus and 2 *cun* lateral to the midline.

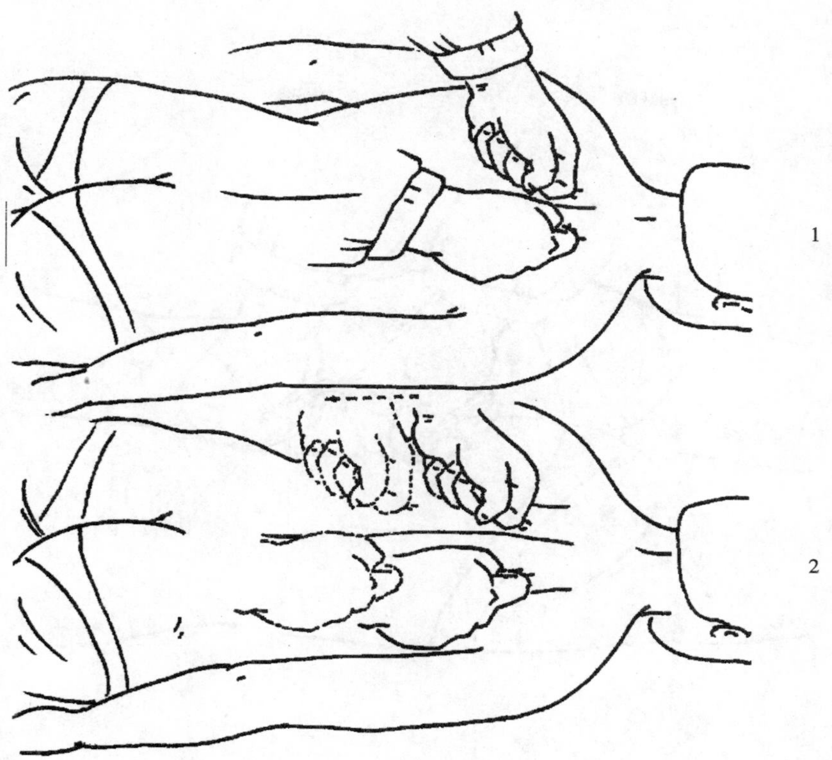

Digital pressing technique on the hypochondrium for reinforcing *qi*.

Manipulation

Place the index finger knuckles of both hands respectively on bilateral Dazhu (BL 11) then press straight downwards along the first line of Bladder Meridian, pass Xinshu (BL 15) and stop at Geshu (BL 17). Repeat the manipulation for 3-5 times.

Points

1. Dazhu (BL 11): At the level of the lower border of the spinous process of the first thoracic vertebra and 1.5 *cun* lateral to the posterior midline.

2. Xinshu (BL 15): At the level of the lower border of the spinous process of the fifth thoracic vertebra and 1.5 *cun* lateral to the posterior midline.

3. Geshu (BL 17): At the level of the lower border of the spinous process of the seventh thoracic vertebra and 1.5 *cun* lateral to the posterior midline.

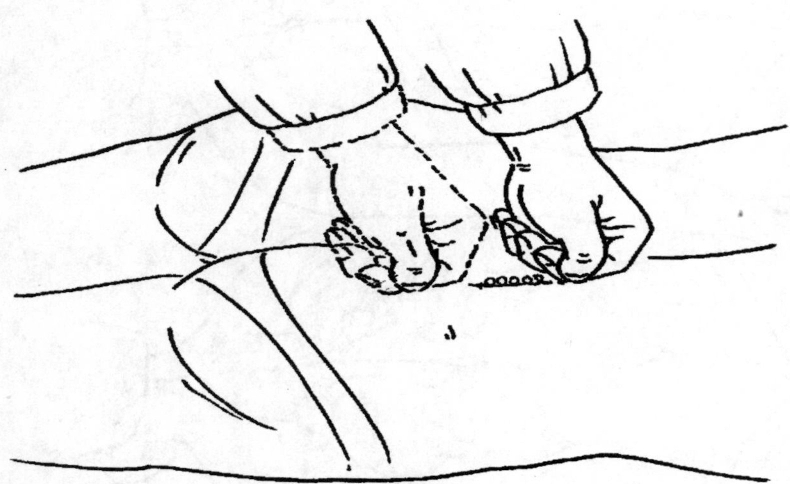

Kneading technique on the lumbosacral region.

Manipulation

Place the back of partially clenched fist on Mingmen (GV 4) and Shenshu (BL 23), then perform kneading technique down the spine to Yaoshu (GV 2) and stop at Baihuanshu (BL 30). Repeat the manipulation for 2-5 minutes.

Points

1. Mingmen (GV 4): Below the spinous process of the second lumbar vertebra.

2. Shenshu (BL 23): At the level of the lower border of the spinous process of the second lumbar vertebra, 1.5 *cun* lateral to the midline.

3. Yaoshu (GV 2): In the hiatus of the sacrum.

4. Baihuanshu (BL 30): At the level of the fourth posterior sacral foramen, 1.5 *cun* lateral to the midline.

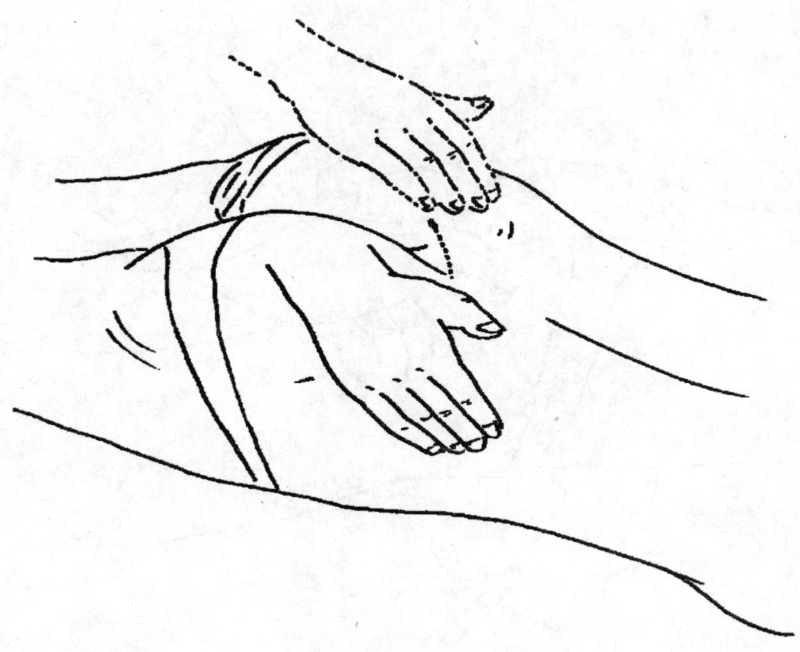

Transverse rubbing technique on the sacrum.

Manipulation

Place one palm on Baohuang (BL 53), rub transversely past Baliao (BL 31-BL 34) and stop at Baohuang (BL 53) on the opposite side. Repeat the manipulation for 3-5 minutes.

Points

1. Baohuang (BL 53): At the level of the second sacral posterior foramen and 3 *cun* lateral to the midline.

2. Baliao (BL 31—BL 34): In the first to fourth posterior sacral foramen of both sides.

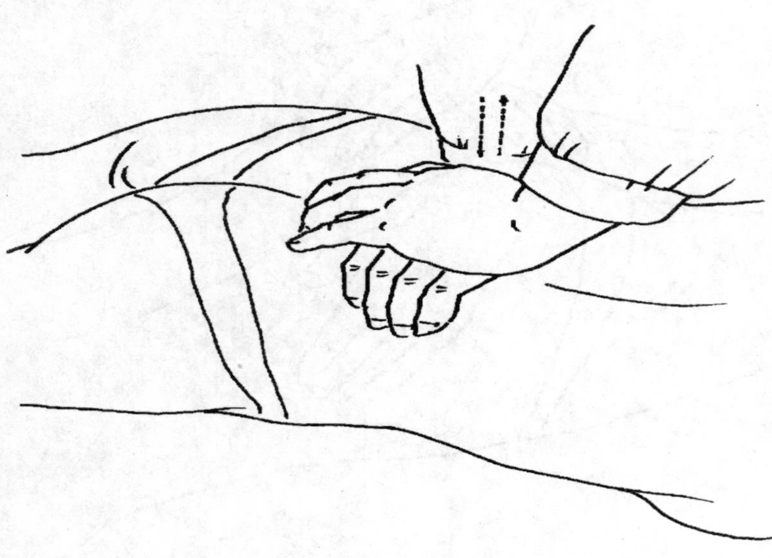

Overlapping palm pressing technique on the lumbar region.

Manipulation

Rub hands together until they are hot, then place one palm on Mingmen (GV 4) and place the other over it. Exert force and develop a rhythm while pressing the point 3-5 times.

Points

Mingmen (GV 4): Below the spinous process of the second lumbar vertebra.

Chronic Pelvic Inflammation

Clinical Manifestations

This disease is characterized by soreness, distention and pain in the lower abdomen and lumbosacral region of female as well as distending pain in the breasts during menstruation, with abnormality in menstrual quantity, color and quality.

Differentiation of syndromes:

A. Retention of damp-heat type: Soreness and pain in the lower abdomen and lumbosacral region, combined with sparse menstrual flow, which is red in color and sticky in quality, or with profuse yellow and thick leukorrhea. Red tongue with yellow and sticky coating, thready wiry or soft rapid pulse.

B. Cold retention and *qi* obstruction type: Cold pain in the lower abdomen, distending pain in the breasts during menstruation, combined with reduced menstrual flow, which is light in color with clots. Deep and tense pulse.

Treatment Principle

Clearing heat and eliminating damp, promoting *qi* and activating blood circulation.

Tuina Techniques

A. Rubbing and pressing techniques on the lower abdomen.
B. Squeezing and pushing techniques on the side of the abdomen.
C. Diagonal rubbing technique on the back.
D. Straight rubbing technique on the lumbar region.
E. Rubbing technique on the buttock.
F. Pushing technique on the lateral aspect of the foot.

Addition or Subtraction Techniques

A. Retention of damp-heat type:

Addition: 1. Diagonal rubbing technique on the hypochondrium. 2. Pressing technique along the medial aspect of the lower leg.

B. Cold retention and *qi* obstruction type:

Addition: 1. Pressing technique along the medial border of the iliac spine. 2.

Pressing technique on Qichong (ST 30). 3. Pressing technique along the medial aspect of the thigh.

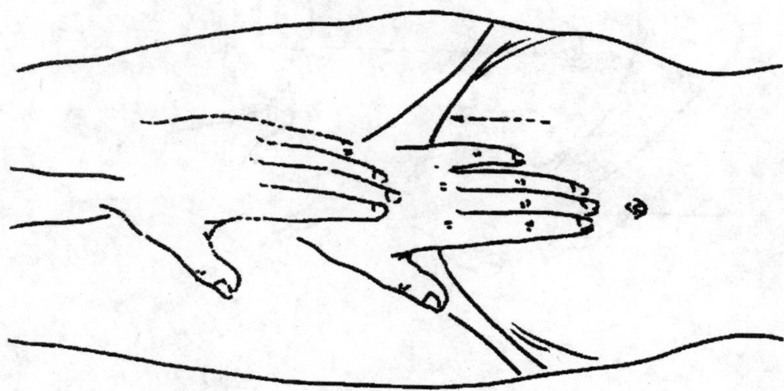

Rubbing and pressing techniques on the lower abdomen.

Manipulation

Place four finger-pulps of one hand on Yinjiao (CV 7), then press and rub straight downwards along the anterior midline to Qugu (CV 2). Repeat the manipulation for 1-2 minutes.

Points

1. Yinjiao (CV 7): 1 *cun* below the center of the umbilicus.
2. Qugu (CV 2): 5 *cun* below the center of the umbilicus.

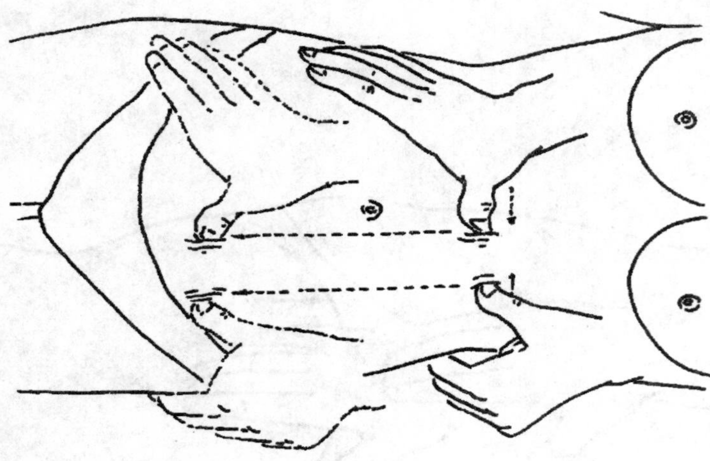

Squeezing and pushing techniques on the side of the abdomen.

Manipulation

With other four fingers on the two sides of the stomach, place two thumbs respectively on Fuai (SP 16) and Shiguan (KI 18), squeeze the abdominal muscle and push straight downwards to Fushe (SP 13) and Qixue (KI 13). Repeat the manipulation for 1-3 minutes.

Points

1. Fuai (SP 16): 3 *cun* directly above the center of the umbilicus and 4 *cun* lateral to the midline.
2. Shiguan (KI 18): 3 *cun* directly above the center of the umbilicus and 0.5 *cun* lateral to the midline.
3. Fushe (SP 13): 3.5 *cun* directly below the center of the umbilicus and 4 *cun* lateral to the midline.
4. Qixue (KI 13): 3 *cun* directly below the center of the umbilicus and 0.5 *cun* lateral to the midline.

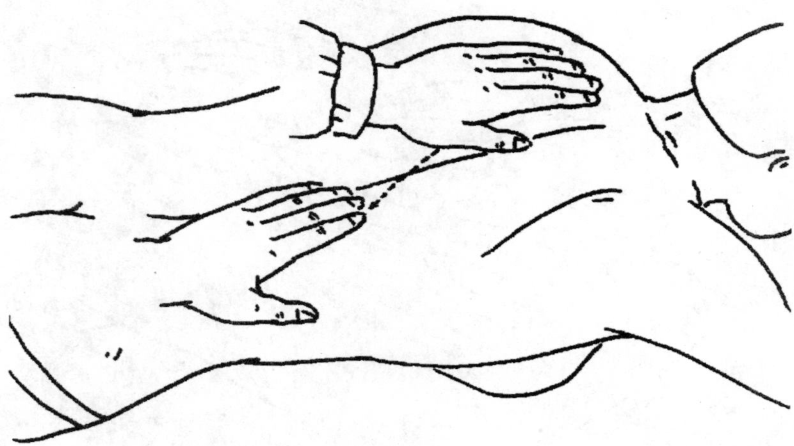

Diagonal rubbing technique on the back.

Manipulation

Place one palm on Jianzhongshu (SI 15), rub diagonally downwards past Jianwaishu (SI 14) and Quyuan (SI 13) and stop at Ganshu (BL 18) on the opposite side. Repeat the manipulation for 5-10 times.

Points

1. Jianzhongshu (SI 15): 2 *cun* lateral to the lower border of the spinous process of the seventh cervical vertebra.

2. Jianwaishu (SI 14): 3 *cun* lateral to the lower border of the spinous process of the first thoracic vertebra.

3. Quyuan (SI 13): On the medial extremity of the suprascapular fossa, at the level of the spinous process of the second thoracic vertebra.

4. Ganshu (BL 18): 1.5 *cun* lateral to the lower border of the spinous process of the ninth thoracic vertebra.

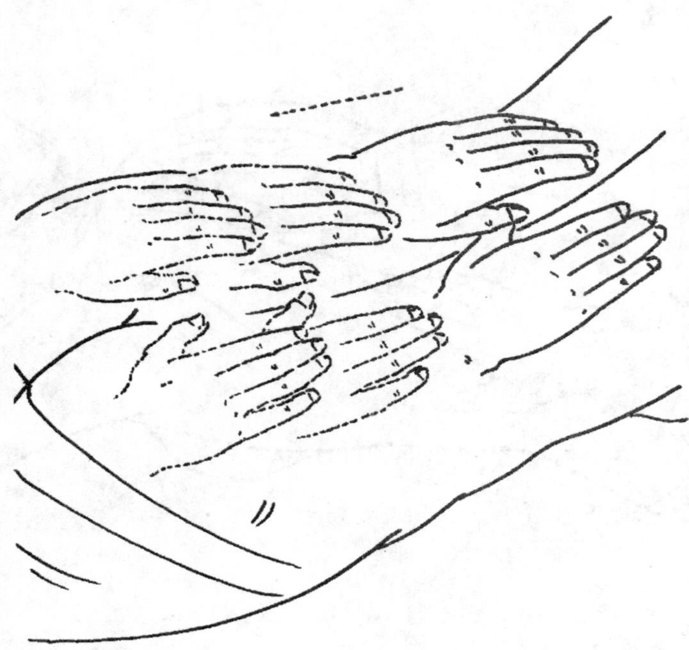

Straight rubbing technique on the lumbar region.

Manipulation

Place four finger-pulps of both hands on Weishu (BL 21) and Weicang (BL 50), rub straight downwards past Shenshu (BL 23), Zhishi (BL 52) and stop at Xiaochangshu (BL 27). Repeat the manipulation 5-15 minutes.

Points

1. Weishu (BL 21): At the level of the lower border of the spinous process of the twelfth thoracic vertebra and 1.5 *cun* lateral to the midline.

2. Weicang (BL 50): 1.5 *cun* lateral to Weishu (BL 21).

3. Shenshu (BL 23): At the level of the lower border of the spinous process of the second lumbar vertebra and 1.5 *cun* lateral to the midline.

4. Zhishi (BL 52): 1.5 *cun* lateral to Shenshu (BL 23).

5. Xiaochangshu (BL 27): At the level of the first posterior sacral foramen and 1.5 *cun* lateral to the midline.

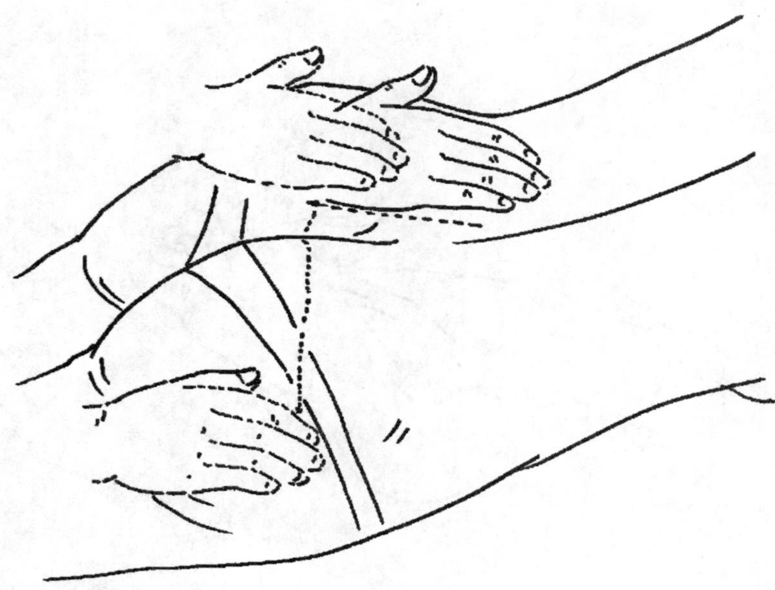

Rubbing technique on the buttock.

Manipulation

Place four finger-pulps of one hand on unilateral Guanyuanshu (BL 26), rub diagonally downwards past Baohuang (BL 53) and stop at Huantiao (GB 30). Repeat the manipulation for 5-10 minutes.

Points

1. Guanyuanshu (BL 26): 1.5 *cun* lateral to the lower border of the spinous process of the fifth lumbar vertebra.

2. Baohuang (BL 53): At the level of the second sacral posterior foramen and 3 *cun* lateral to the midline.

3. Huantiao (GB 30): At the junction of the lateral 1/3 and medial 2/3 of the distance between the great trochanter and the hiatus of the sacrum.

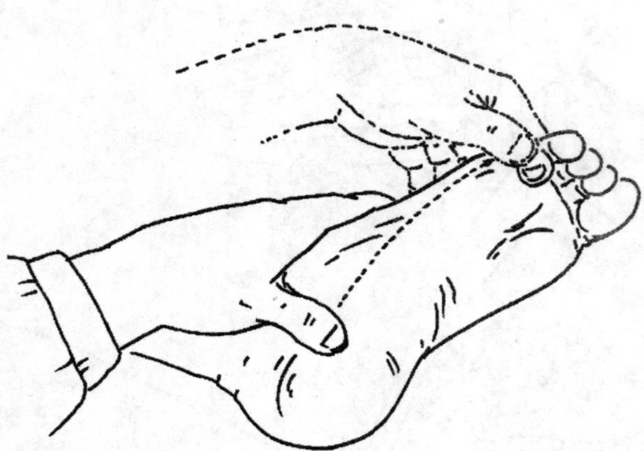

Pushing technique on the lateral aspect of the foot.

Manipulation

Place one thumb on Pucan (BL 61) and grip the back of the foot with other four fingers. Push along the lateral margin of the foot (Bladder Meridian) to Zhiyin (BL 67), then press the distal section of the little toe to bend it down. Repeat the manipulation 2-5 minutes.

Points

1. Pucan (BL 61):Directly below the depression between the external malleolus and tendo calcaneus, at the junction of red and white skin.

2. Zhiyin (BL 67): On the lateral side of the small toe, about 0.1 *cun* posterior to the corner of the nail.

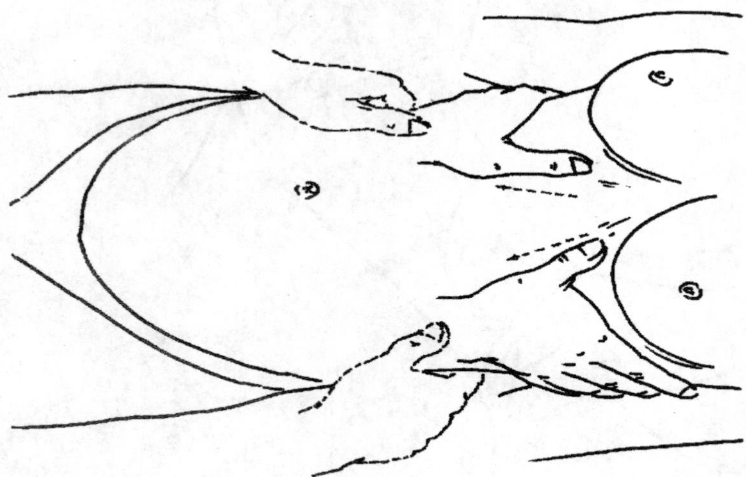

Diagonal rubbing technique on the hypochondrium.

Manipulation

Place two thumbs on Burong (ST 19) and Chengman (ST 20), then rub along the lower border of rib cage diagonally and stop at both sides of Zhangmen (LR 13). Repeat the manipulation for 3-5 minutes.

Points

1. Burong (ST 19): 6 *cun* above the center of the umbilicus and 2 *cun* lateral to the midline.

2. Chengman (ST 20): 5 *cun* above the center of the umbilicus and 2 *cun* lateral to the midline.

3. Zhangmen (LR 13): On the lateral side of the abdomen, below the free end of the eleventh floating rib.

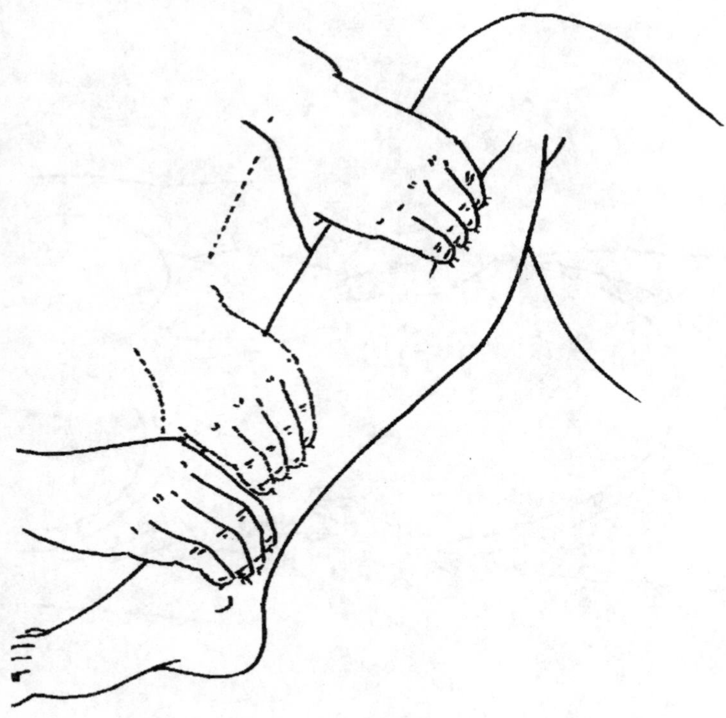

Pressing technique along the medial aspect of the lower leg.

Manipulation

Place four fingertips of one hand on Yinlingquan (SP 9), then press and knead downwards along the medial border of the tibia to Sanyinjiao (SP 6). At the same time, place other four fingertips on Taixi (KI 3) and knead the point. Repeat the manipulation for 1-3 minutes.

Points

1. Yinlingquan (SP 9): On the lower border of the medial condyle of the tibia, in the depression on the medial border of the tibia.

2. Sanyinjiao (SP 6): 3 *cun* directly above the tip of the medial malleolus, on the posterior border of the medial aspect of the tibia.

3. Taixi (KI 3): In the depression between the medial malleolus and tendo calcaneus.

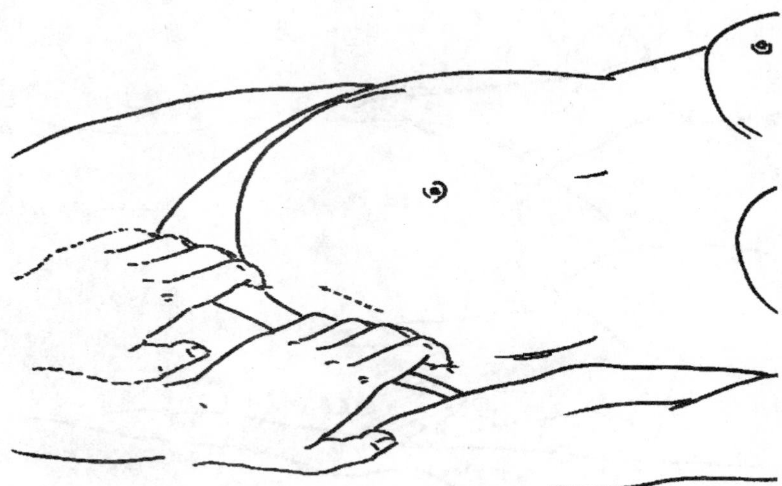

Pressing technique along the medial border of the iliac bone.

Manipulation

Place four fingertips on Wushu (GB 27) located on the side of the ilium, and then press and push down to Qichong (ST 30). Repeat the manipulation for 1-2 minutes.

Points

1. Wushu (GB 27): 0.5 *cun* anterior to the anterior superior iliac spine.
2. Qichong (ST 30): 5 *cun* directly below the center of the umbilicus and 2 *cun* lateral to the anterior midline.

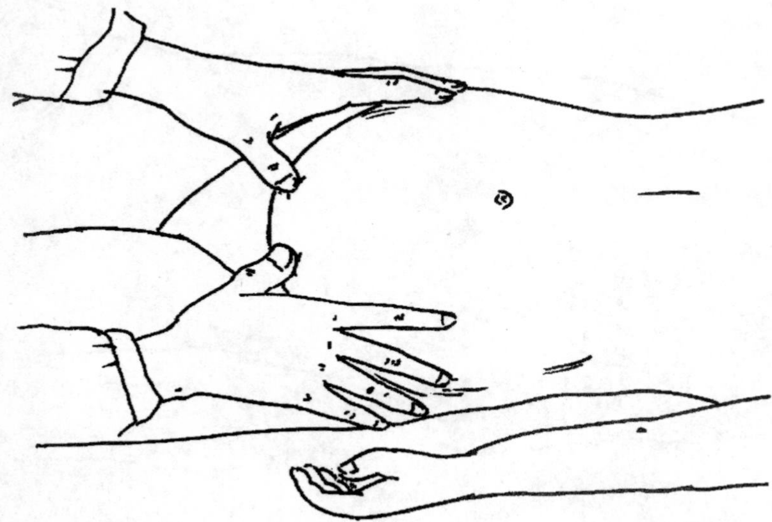

Pressing technique on Qichong (ST 30).

Manipulation

Place two thumbs on bilateral Qichong (ST 30) and apply pressure to the points for 1-3 times, each time lasts 10-30 seconds, and then release the thumbs.

Points

Qichong (ST 30): 5 *cun* directly below the center of the umbilicus and 2 *cun* lateral to the midline.

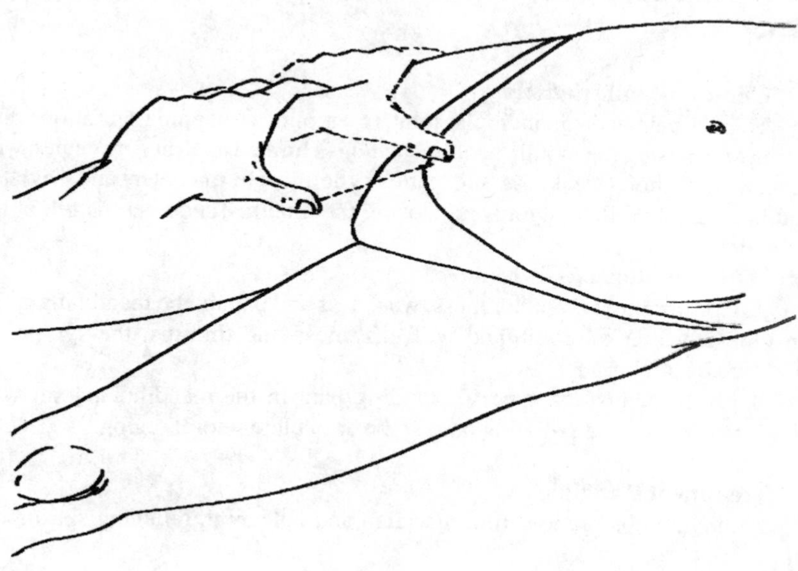

Pressing technique along the medial aspect of the thigh.

Manipulation

Place a thumb on Yinlian (LR 11) and grip the back of leg with other four fingers. Press the point forcefully for 3-5 times, each time lasts 15-30 seconds. Then push up to Qichong (ST 30) and then press the point 1-3 times, each time lasts 30-60 seconds.

Points

1. Yinlian (LR 11): 2 *cun* lateral and 2 *cun* below the midpoint of the upper margin of the pubic bone.

2. Qichong (ST 30): 5 *cun* directly below the center of the umbilicus and 2 *cun* lateral to the midline.

Temporomandibular Joint Syndrome

Clinical Manifestations

There is pain in the mandibular joint, resembling a snapping sensation while opening and closing the mouth. Mouth opening is limited to a varying degree with soreness, distention, weakness and pain of the muscle masseter, and deviated mandibular joint while opening and closing the mouth. Tenderness is felt at the joint region.

Differentiation of syndromes:

A. Consumption type: Soreness, weakness and pain in the mandibular joint with repeated attacks, combined with dizziness and tinnitus, the symptoms aggravated by strain.

B. Blood stagnation type: Distending pain in the mandibular joint with obvious tenderness and radiating pain at the auriculotemporal region.

Treatment Principle

Removing obstruction from meridian and collateral, relieving spasm and pain.

Tuina Techniques

A. Facial circular kneading and nipping techniques.

B. Pressing technique on Shangguan (GB 3) and Xiaguan (ST 7).

C. Pushing technique on Jiache (ST 6).

D. Separate pushing technique on the occipital region.

E. Pressing technique on Wangu (GB 12).

F. Kneading technique on Hegu (LI 4).

Addition or Subtraction Techniques

A. Consumption type:

Addition: 1. Separate pushing technique on the forehead. 2. Improving hearing ability technique.

B. Blood stagnation type:

Addition: 1. Pushing technique on the lateral aspect of the head. 2. Opposite pressing technique on the head. 3. Pinching technique on the cervical muscles.

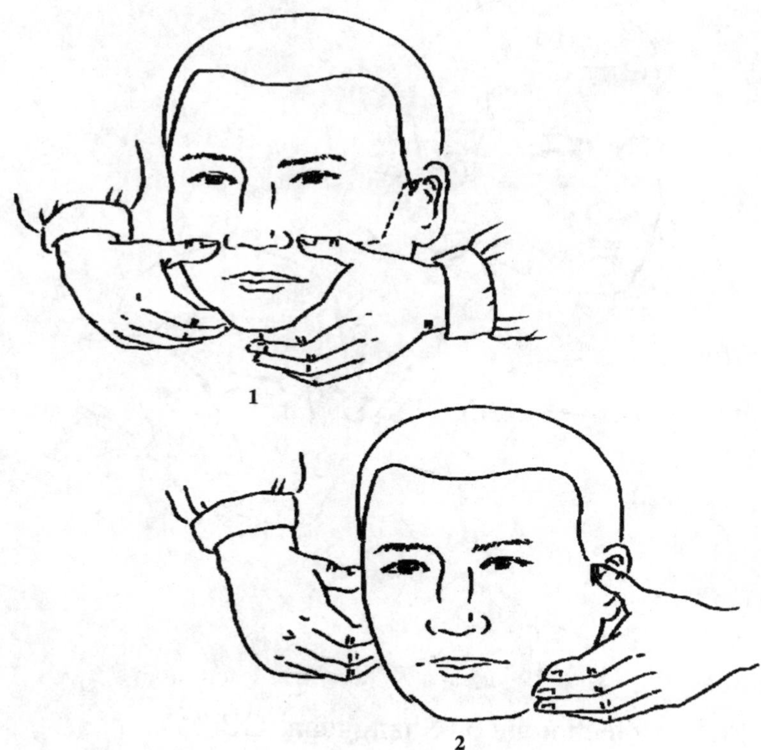

Facial circular kneading and nipping techniques.

Manipulation

Place two thumbs respectively on bilateral Yingxiang (LI 20), first apply pressing and nipping techniques, then rubbing and pushing along the lower border of the maxilla past Quanliao (SI 18), Xiaguan (ST 7), and stop at Ermen (TE 21). Repeat the manipulation for 1-3 minutes.

Points

1. Yingxiang (LI 20): In the nasolabial groove, at the level of the midpoint of the lateral border of ala nasi.

2. Quanliao (SI 18): Directly below the outer canthus, in the depression on the lower border of zygoma.

3. Xiaguan (ST 7): At the lower border of the zygomatic arch, in the depression anterior to the condyloid process of the mandible.

4. Ermen (TE 21): In the depression anterior to the supratragic notch and slightly superior to the condyloid process of the mandible.

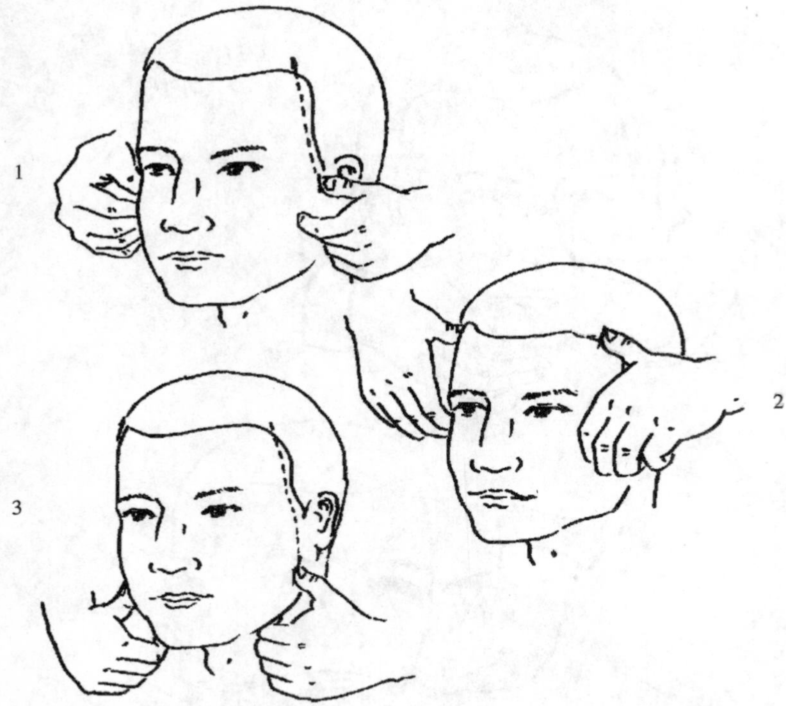

Pressing technique on Shangguan (GB 3) and Xiaguan (ST 7).

Manipulation

Place two thumbs and index fingertips respectively on bilateral Shangguan (GB 3) and Xiaguan (ST 7), massage in kneading method for 1-3 minutes. Then let the thumbs push upwards to Touwei (ST 8), and the index fingers push downwards to Jiache (ST 6). Repeat the pushing technique for 1-2 minutes.

Points

1. Shangguan (GB 3): On the upper border of the zygomatic arch, in the depression directly above Xiaguan (ST 7).

2. Xiaguan (ST 7): At the lower border of the zygomatic arch, in the depression anterior to the condyloid process of the mandible.

3. Touwei (ST 8): 0.5 *cun* within the anterior hairline at the corner of the forehead, 4.5 *cun* lateral to the midline.

4. Jiache (ST 6): One finger-breadth anterior and superior to the lower angle of the mandible where m. masseter attaches at the prominence of the muscle when the teeth are clenched.

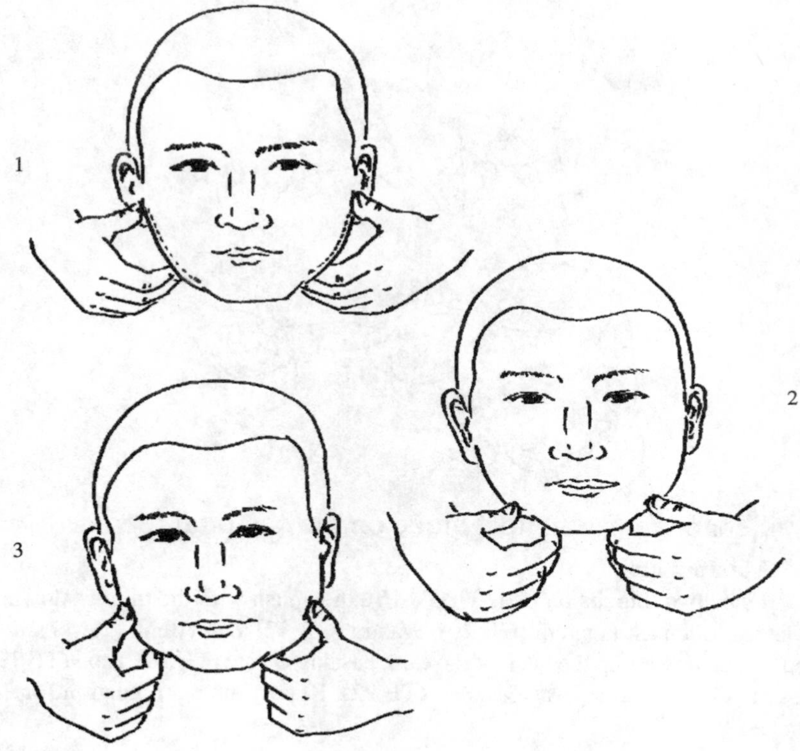

Pushing technique on Jiache (ST 6).

Manipulation

Place two thumbs respectively on bilateral Tinghui (GB 2), then push downwards along the lateral border of the mandibula past Jiache (ST 6) and stop at Daying (ST 5). Repeat the massage 3-5 minutes. Then knead Jiache (ST 6) for 1-2 minutes.

Points

1. Tinghui (GB 2): Anterior to the intertragic notch, at the posterior border of the condyloid process of the mandible. The point is located with the mouth open.

2. Jiache (ST 6): One finger-breadth anterior and superior to the lower angle of the mandible where m. masseter attaches at the prominence of the muscle when the teeth are clenched.

3. Daying (ST 5): In the depression, 1.3 *cun* anterior to the angle of mandible.

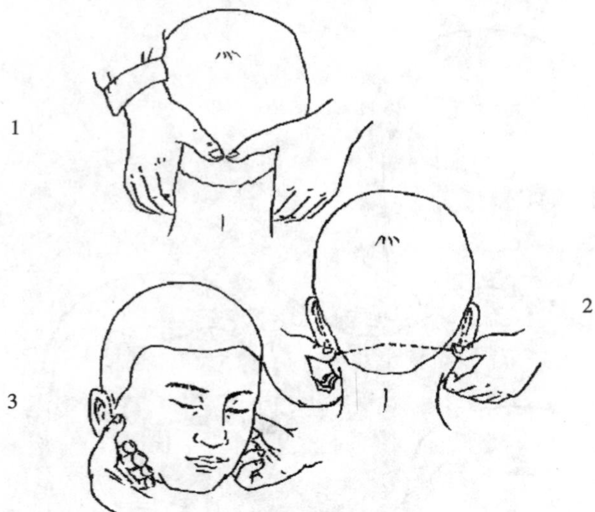

Separate pushing technique on the occipital region.

Manipulation

Place two thumbs on Fengfu (GV 16), then push with the thumbs down to the lateral side past Fengchi (GB 20), Wangu (GB 12) and Yifeng (TE 17), then keep on pushing along the back of the ears, passing Qimai (TE 18), Luxi (TE 19), Jiaosun (TE 20) and stop at Erheliao (TE 22). Repeat the manipulation for 2-3 minutes.

Points

1. Fengfu (GV 16): 1 *cun* directly above the midpoint of the posterior hairline.
2. Fengchi (GB 20): In the depression between the upper portion of m. Sternocleidomastoideus and m. trapezius, on the same level with Fengfu (GV 16).
3. Wangu (GB 12): In the depression posterior and inferior to the mastoid process.
4. Yifeng (TE 17): Posterior to the lobule of the ear, in the depression between the mandible and mastoid process.
5. Qimai (TE 18): In the center of the mastoid process, at the junction of the middle and lower third of the curve formed by Yifeng (TE 17) and Jiaosun (TE 20) posterior to the helix.
6. Luxi (TE 19): Posterior to the ear, at the junction of the upper and middle third of the curve formed by Yifeng (TE 17) and Jiaosun (TE 20) behind the helix.
7. Jiaosun (TE 20): Directly above the ear apex, within the hairline.
8. Erheliao (TE 22): Anterior and superior to Ermen (TE 21), at the level with the root of the auricle, on the posterior border of the hairline of the temple where the superficial temporal artery passes.

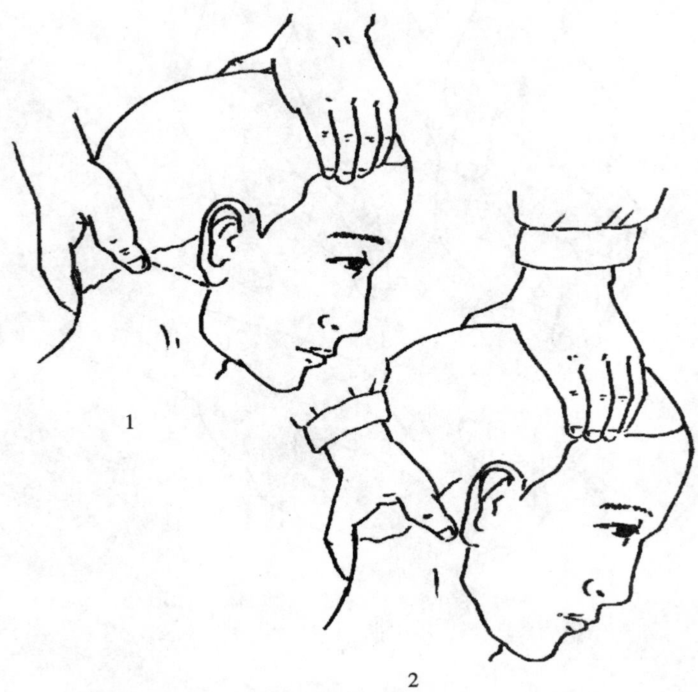

Pressing technique on Wangu (GB 12).

Manipulation

Place one thumb on unilateral Wangu (GB 12), press and knead the point for 1-2 minutes. Then let the thumb push to Yifeng (TE 17). Repeat the manipulation 1-2 minutes.

Points

1. Wangu (GB 12): In the depression posterior and inferior to the mastoid process.

2. Yifeng (TE 17): Posterior to the lobule of the ear, in the depression between the mandible and mastoid process.

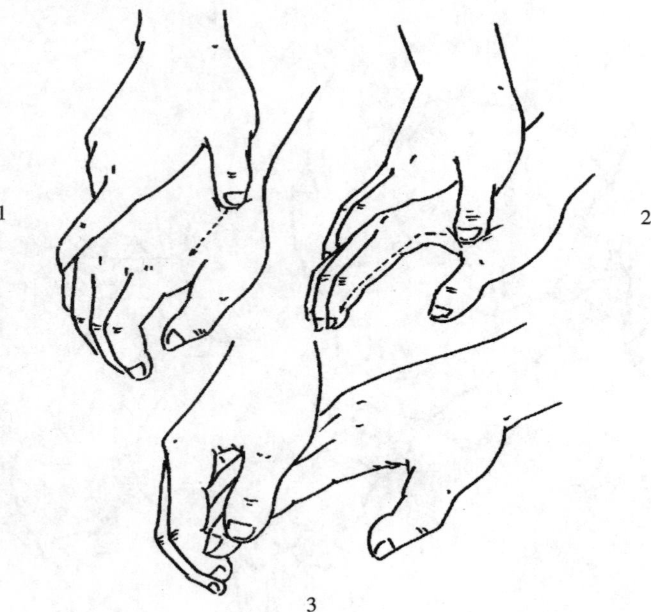

Kneading technique on Hegu (LI 4).

Manipulation

Place a thumb on Yangxi (LI 5) located at the wrist, lay other four fingers at the side of the hand. Push downwards with the thumb from Yangxi (LI 5) to Hegu (LI 4) and knead the point for 10-30 seconds, then push along the side of the index finger (large intestine meridian) to Shangyang (LI 1). Repeat the manipulation for 3-5 times.

Points

1. Yangxi (LI 5): On the radial side of the wrist, in the depression between the tendons of m. extensor pollicis longus and brevis.

2. Hegu (LI 4): On the dorsum of the hand, between the first and second metacarpal bones, approximately in the middle of the second metacarpal bone on the radial side.

3. Shangyang (LI 1): On the radial side of the index finger, about 0.1 *cun* posterior to the corner of the nail.

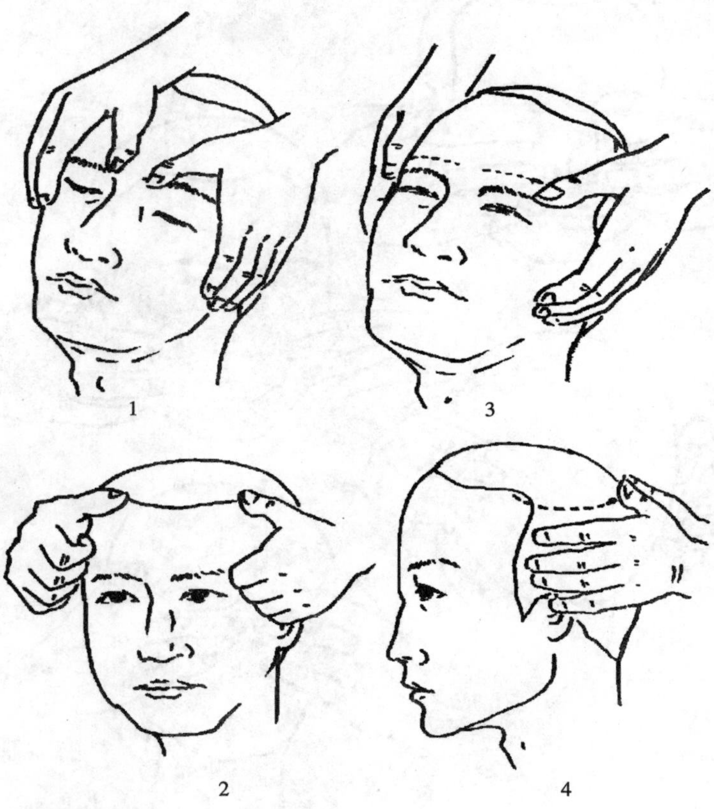

Separate pushing technique on the forehead.

Manipulation

Place two thumbs on the forehead center, then push to the sides of the forehead for 1-3 minutes. Then place two thumbs respectively on Touwei (ST 8), and rub backward to Houding (GV 19). Repeat the massage 1-2 minutes.

Points

1. Touwei (ST 8): 0.5 *cun* within the anterior hairline at the corner of the forehead, 4.5 *cun* lateral to the midline.

2. Houding (GV 19): On the midline of the head, 5.5 *cun* directly above the posterior hairline.

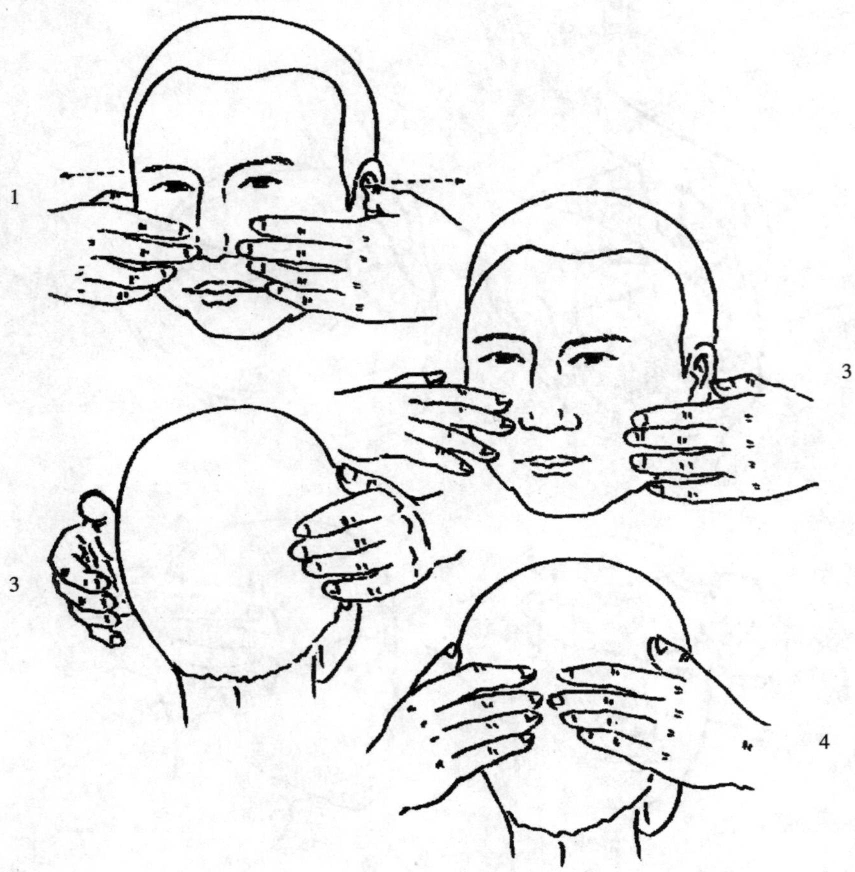

Improving hearing ability technique.

Manipulation

1. Cover ear holes with two thumbs and instruct the patient to inhale deeply and close the mouth, restraining temporarily from exhaling, immediately place the middle finger of each hand on the wings of nose to close the nostrils for a while, then release the thumbs and middle fingers away from the ears and nose, at the same time instruct the patient to exhale deeply. Repeat this manipulation for 3-5 times.

2. Place the palms of both hands firmly against the auricle of each ear, while lay the four fingers of both hands on the occipital bone. Use middle fingers to gently tap the back of head so that there will be a thumping sound in the patient's ears. Repeat the tapping 36 times.

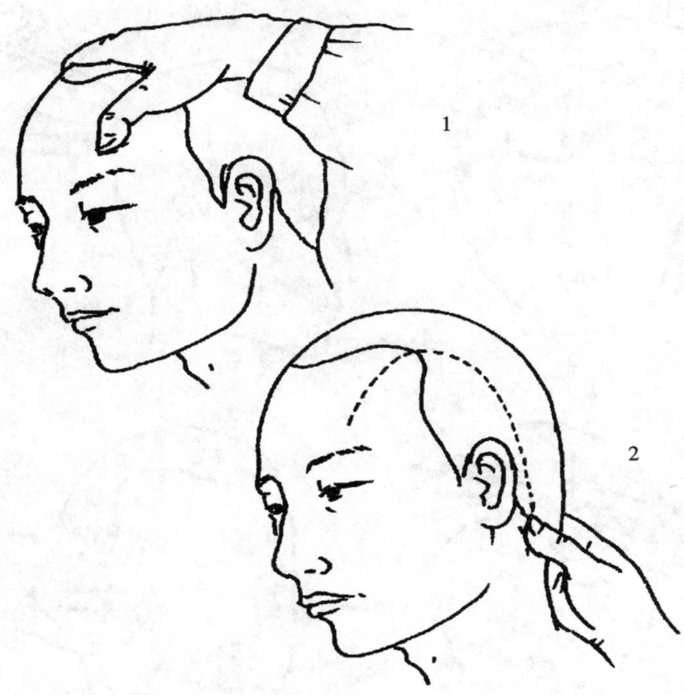

Pushing technique on the lateral aspect of the head.

Manipulation

Place a thumb on Yangbai (GB 14), then push upwards, backwards and downwards along the gallbladder meridian as shown in figure 2 past Benshen (GB 13) and stop at Wangu (GB 12). Repeat the manipulation for 2-3 minutes.

Points

1. Yangbai (GB 14): On the forehead, 1 *cun* directly above the midpoint of the eyebrow.

2. Benshen (GB 13): 0.5 *cun* within the hairline of the forehead, 3 *cun* lateral to the midline.

3. Wangu (GB 12): In the depression posterior and inferior to the mastoid process.

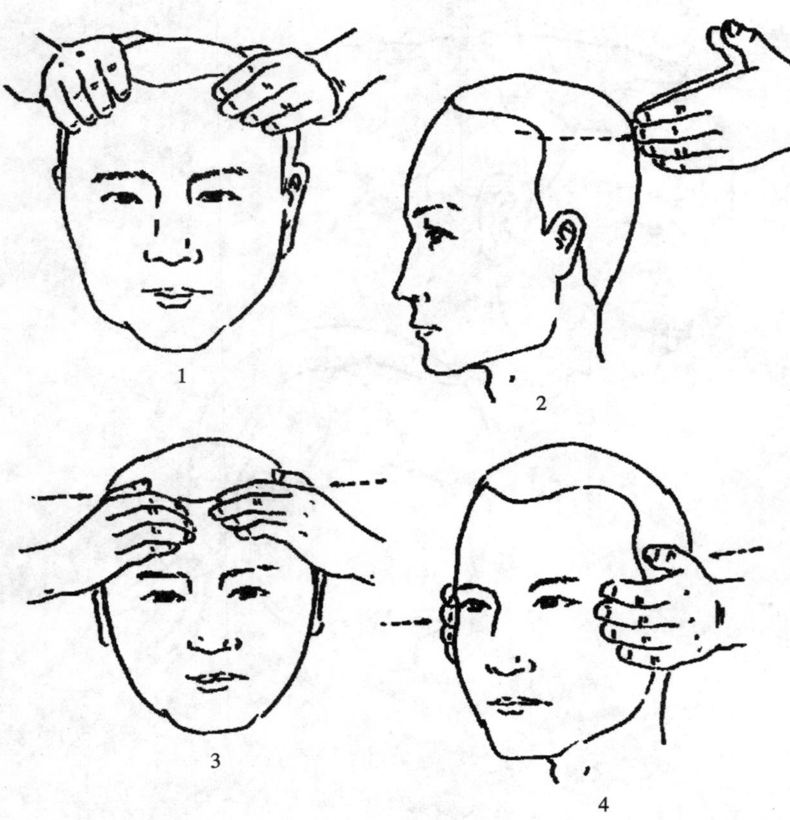

Opposite pressing technique on the head .

Manipulation

1. Place four finger-pulps of each hand on Touwei (ST 8) located at the side of the forehead, then rub backward to Houding (GV 19), repeat it 1-3 minutes.

2. Let the palms press the temple regions vigorously, then the ears for 1-3 minutes.

Points

1. Touwei (ST 8): 0.5 *cun* within the anterior hairline at the corner of the forehead, 4.5 *cun* lateral to the midline.

2. Houding (GV 19): On the midline of the head, 5.5 *cun* directly above the posterior hairline.

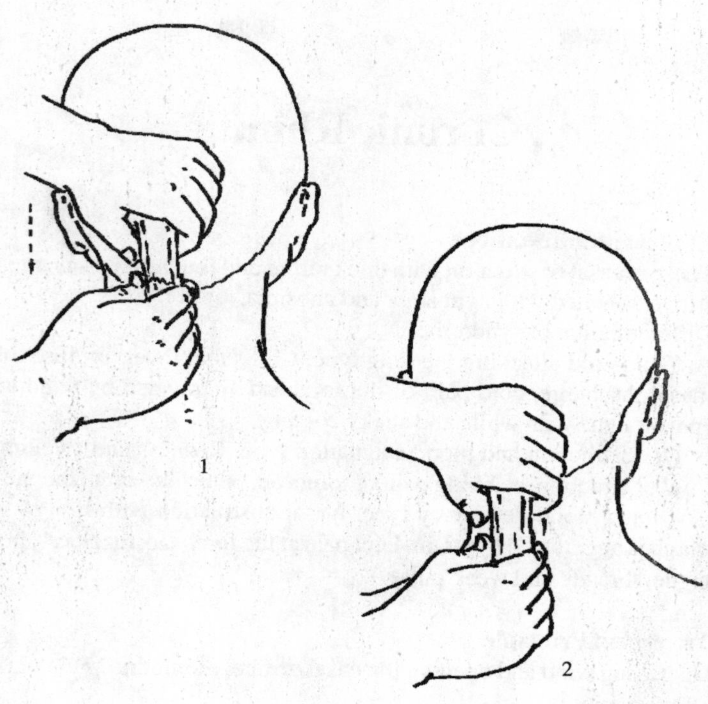

Pinching technique on the cervical muscles.

Manipulation

Place finger tips of both hands on unilateral Fengchi (GB 20), the thumbs on the lateral side of the neck muscle and the four fingers on the medial pinch and pull up the neck muscle starting from Fengchi (GB 20) down to Jianzhongshu (SI 15). Repeat the manipulation respectively for 1-2 minutes on the left side and right side of the neck.

Points

1. Fengchi (GB 20): In the depression between the upper portion of m. sternocleidomastoideus and m. trapezius, on the same level with Fengfu (GV 16).

2. Jianzhongshu (SI 15): 2 *cun* lateral to the lower border of the spinous process of the seventh cervical vertebra.

Chronic Rhinitis

Clinical Manifestations

There is nasal obstruction with thick turbid and foul nasal discharge, or post nasal drip, associated with hyposmia and anosmia.

Differentiation of syndromes:

A. Wind-cold attacking the lung type: Chills and fever, profuse thick and turbid nasal discharge, cold pain of the forehead aggravated by wind and cold attack, pale tongue with white and sticky coating.

B. *Qi* obstruction and blood stagnation type: Redness and swelling of the nose, nasal obstruction, stabbing pain of forehead, petechiae at the tongue border.

C. *Qi* and blood deficiency type: Nasal obstruction with loss of sense of smell which is aggravated by strain. Dull pain at the forehead, dizziness, insomnia, pale tongue, thready and weak pulse.

Treatment Principle

Dispelling wind and opening the nasal orifice, promoting *qi* circulation and restore vital energy.

Tuina Techniques

A. Facial circular kneading and nipping techniques.

B. Nipping technique on Sibai (ST 2).

C. Separate pushing technique on the occipital region.

D. Nipping technique on Sishencong (Ex-HN 1).

E. Kneading technique on Hegu (LI 4).

Addition or Subtraction Techniques

A. Wind-cold attacking the lung type:

Addition: 1. Stationary circular pressing technique on Fengchi (GB 20). 2. Pressing technique on Zhongfu (LU 1) and Yunmen (LU 2).

B. *Qi* obstruction and blood stagnation type:

Addition: 1. Stationary circular pressing technique on Taiyang (Ex-HN 5). 2. Pressing technique on Juliao (ST 3).

C. *Qi* and blood deficiency type:

Addition: 1. Separate pushing technique on the forehead. 2. Pressing technique on Wangu (GB 12).

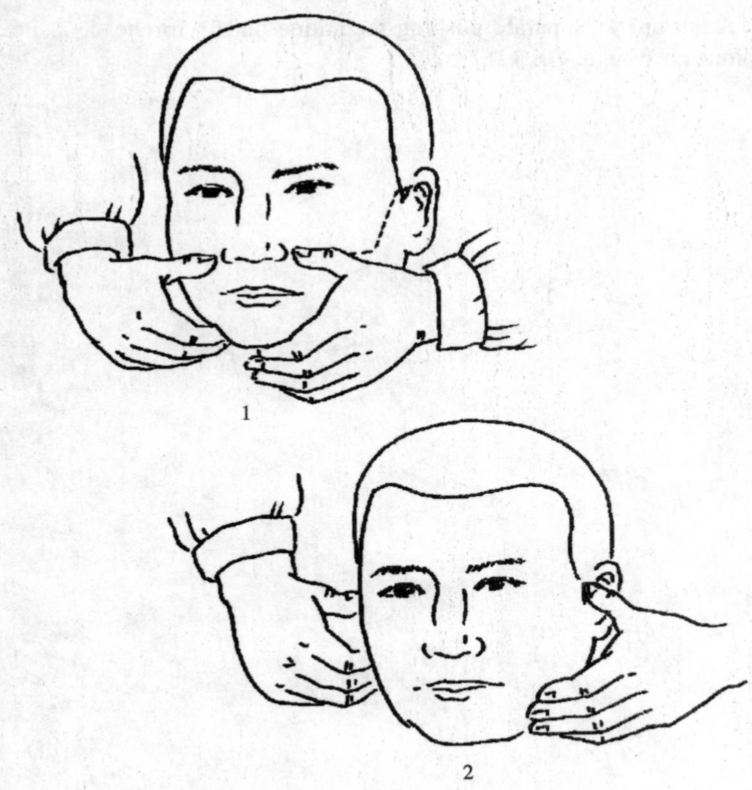

1

2

Facial circular kneading and nipping techniques.

Manipulation

Place two thumbs on Yingxiang (LI 20) of the face, from where first apply pressing and nipping techniques, then rub and push along the lower border of the maxilla past Quanliao (SI 18), Xiaguan (ST 7) and stop at Ermen (TE 21). Repeat the manipulation for 1-3 minutes.

Points

1. Yingxiang (LI 20): In the nasolabial groove, at the level of the midpoint of the lateral border of ala nasi.

2. Quanliao (SI 18): Directly below the outer canthus, in the depression on the lower border of zygoma.

3. Xiaguan (ST 7): At the lower border of the zygomatic arch, in the depression anterior to the condyloid process of the mandible.

4. Ermen (TE 21): In the depression anterior to the supratragic notch and slightly superior to the condyloid process of the mandible.